Tardive Dyskinesia

and
Related Involuntary
Movement Disorders

The Long-Term Effects of
Antipsychotic Drugs

Edited by

Joseph DeVeaugh-Geiss

John Wright • PSG Inc
Boston   Bristol   London
1982

Library of Congress Cataloging in Publication Data
Main entry under title:

Tardive dyskinesia and related involuntary
movement disorders.

Bibliography: p.
Includes index .
1. Tardive dyskinesia. 2. Psychotropic
drugs--Side effects. I. DeVeaugh-Geiss,
Joseph, 1946-   . [DNLM: 1. Dyskinesia,
Drug-induced--Congresses. 2. Tranquilizing
agents, Major--Adverse effects--
Congresses. WL
390 T182 1979-80]
RC394.T37T36   616.8'3   81-16387
ISBN 0-7236-7006-4   AACR2

Published by:
John Wright • PSG Inc, 545 Great Road, Littleton,
Massachusetts 01460, U.S.A.
John Wright & Sons Ltd, 42–44 Triangle West,
Bristol BS8 1EX, England

Medicine is an ever-changing science. As new research and clinical experience broaden our knowledge, changes in treatment and drug therapy are required. The editor and the publisher of this work have made every effort to ensure that the treatment and drug dosage schedules herein are accurate and in accord with the standards accepted at the time of publication. Readers are advised, however, to check the product information sheet included in the package of each drug they plan to administer to be certain that changes have not been made in the recommended dose or in the indications and contraindications for administration. This recommendation is of particular importance in regard to new or infrequently used drugs.

Printed in Great Britain by John Wright & Sons (Printing) Ltd.
at The Stonebridge Press, Bristol.

International Standard Book Number: 0-7236-7006-4

Library of Congress Catalog Card Number: 81-16387

CONTRIBUTORS

Murray Alpert, PhD
Professor, Director of Psychology
New York University Medical Center
New York, New York

Irwin Birnbaum, LLB
Lecturer in Legal Medicine
State University of New York
  Upstate Medical Center
Practicing Attorney
Syracuse, New York

Anthony J. Blowers, PhD
University of Sussex
Sussex, England

Richard L. Borison, MD, PhD
Associate Professor of Psychiatry,
  Neurology, and Pharmacology
Medical College of Georgia
Augusta, Georgia

Eric D. Caine, MD
Assistant Professor of Psychiatry
  and Neurology
University of Rochester School of
  Medicine and Dentistry
Rochester, New York

Daniel E. Casey, MD
Research Associate, Departments of
  Medical Research and Psychiatry
Portland Veterans Administration
  Hospital
Associate Professor of Psychiatry
University of Oregon Health
  Sciences Center
Portland, Oregon

Guy Chouinard, MD, MSc
Associate Professor of Psychiatry
McGill University
Psychiatrist
Hôpital Louis-H. Lafontaine and
  Allan Memorial Institute
Montreal, Quebec, Canada

George E. Crane, MD
Clinical Professor of Psychiatry
University of North Dakota
  School of Medicine
Grand Forks, North Dakota

Robert W. Daly, MD
Professor of Psychiatry
State University of New York
  Upstate Medical Center
Syracuse, New York

Bruce Dearing, PhD, LLD
University Professor of Humanities
  in Medicine
State University of New York
Syracuse, New York

Joseph DeVeaugh-Geiss, MD
Assistant Professor of Psychiatry
Adjunct Assistant Professor of
  Neurology
State University of New York
  Upstate Medical Center
Director, Tardive Dyskinesia Clinic
Syracuse Veterans Administration
  Medical Center
Syracuse, New York

Bruce I. Diamond, PhD
Associate Professor of Psychiatry
  and Neurology
Medical College of Georgia
Augusta, Georgia

Arnold J. Friedhoff, MD
Professor of Psychiatry
Director, Millhauser Laboratories
New York University School of
  Medicine
New York, New York

Alan J. Gelenberg, MD
Assistant Professor of Psychiatry
Harvard Medical School
Chief, Special Studies Clinic
Massachusetts General Hospital
Boston, Massachusetts

iv

Jes Gerlach, MD
Head, Department H
Sct. Hans Hospital
Roskilde, Denmark

Richard G. Giaccio, MD
Staff Psychiatrist and Neurologist
Hutchings Psychiatric Center
Syracuse, New York

John H. Growdon, MD
Assistant Professor of Neurology
Tufts University School of Medicine
Boston, Massachusetts

John M. Kane, MD
Director, Psychiatric Research
Long Island Jewish-Hillside Medical
    Center
Glen Oaks, New York

Luciano M. Modesti, MD
Associate Professor of Neurosurgery
State University of New York
    Upstate Medical Center
Syracuse, New York

Donald M. Pirodsky, MD
Assistant Professor of Psychiatry
State University of New York
    Upstate Medical Center
Director, Consultation-Liaison Service
Syracuse Veterans Administration
    Medical Center
Syracuse, New York

James M. Smith, PhD
Director for Quality Assurance
Hudson River Psychiatric Center
Poughkeepsie, New York
Adjunct Assistant Professor of
    Psychiatry
New York University Medical Center
New York, New York

Joanne D. Wojcik, RN, MS
Assistant Chief
Special Studies Clinic
Erich Lindemann Mental Health
    Center and Massachusetts
    General Hospital
Boston, Massachusetts

Richard J. Wurtman, MD
Professor of Neuroendocrine
    Regulation
Massachusetts Institute of Technology
Cambridge, Massachusetts

Steven H. Zeisel, MD, PhD
Research Associate
Department of Nutrition and
    Food Science
Massachusetts Institute of Technology
Cambridge, Massachusetts

CONTENTS

PREFACE

During the past three decades, the practice of psychiatry has been profoundly influenced by the introduction of a large number of psychoactive drugs which are now used in the treatment of the commonly recognized major psychiatric syndromes. This *pharmacologic revolution* has been credited with reducing the populations of mental hospitals worldwide, with alleviating or reducing the disability and suffering of mental patients, and with returning many patients to their homes and communities where they may lead semi-autonomous and more productive lives.

While the benefits of drug therapies to patients and society may be exaggerated by some, there is no doubt that these drugs confer many benefits, and few psychiatrists would wish to return to the psychiatric practices of the prepharmacologic era. Unfortunately, the harmful effects of the antipsychotic (neuroleptic) drugs were unknown when chlorpromazine was introduced in 1952, and when these drugs were embraced with such enthusiasm that they were sometimes used excessively and inappropriately. One result of the large scale use of these drugs was that the movement disorder of tardive dyskinesia occurred in a substantial number of patients.

It is now clear that neuroleptic drugs cause tardive dyskinesia and that this syndrome has become the most serious and troublesome complication of antipsychotic drug therapy. This movement disorder has created a challenge for the practitioner and the patient, who must now choose — as is often the case in medical and moral dilemmas — between two evils: the disability of a chronic psychosis or the disability of a treatment-induced movement disorder that is untreatable. Tardive dyskinesia has also created a challenge to the psychiatrist in the way of malpractice litigation. As a result, many practitioners have become uncertain about what to do when faced with the decision of whether, and how, to treat psychotic patients.

Because of these serious concerns, and with the belief that the accumulated knowledge of the past decade could bring some rationality to discussions of these problems, I organized two symposia devoted entirely to tardive dyskinesia and related disorders. These symposia took place in Syracuse, New York, in 1979 and 1980, and consisted of four days of presentations by, and interactions among, experts from several disciplines. The symposia were considered to be rewarding for those who participated, and it was generally felt that what we accomplished would be useful to others and should be published. The final result is this book, in which I have attempted to synthesize the proceedings of those four days. I sincerely hope this text will prove to be clinically useful and, moreover, that it may help to reduce the incidence of iatrogenic disease among psychiatric patients.

Essentially, all portions of this book were originally presented orally and were transcribed for publication from audiotapes. Some chapters have been revised and updated by the authors, while others appear, with minor editorial changes, much as they were presented. The style of presentation, therefore, varies from one chapter to another. I hope that this will not be too distracting to the reader. I have attempted to integrate the materials and eliminate duplication where this could be accomplished without altering the content of the original presentations. However, there are some areas of overlapping as would be expected with such a specific and limited subject. I apologize for this redundancy, although I believe that reiteration and reinforcement of certain central concepts is often desirable. I wish to thank each of the participants for their conscientious cooperation and excellent contribution, and to credit them for the strengths of this book. Its weaknesses are my responsibility. I also thank Diane Ryan and Barbara Svoboda for transcribing the original audiotapes, and Janine Deferio for typing the final manuscript. Last, but not least, I thank my wife and family for supporting me through the arduous tasks of organizing and conducting the two symposia and of assembling and editing the materials for this publication, for without their patience and assistance, these endeavors could not have succeeded.

Joseph DeVeaugh-Geiss
Syracuse, New York
February, 1981

1 Tardive Dyskinesia: Phenomenology, Pathophysiology, and Pharmacology

Joseph DeVeaugh-Geiss

Tardive dyskinesia is a choreiform, involuntary movement disorder resembling Huntington's disease. Both are characterized by incessant, rhythmic involuntary movements, and these are generally hyperkinetic movement disorders in contrast to Parkinson's disease, in which one of the main features is reduction of movement (hypokinesia). The most common form of tardive dyskinesia involves the orofacial musculature and may manifest as blepharospasm, grimacing, masticatory movements, lip-pursing, puffing of the cheeks, and licking or protrusion of the tongue. Frequently, choreoathetosis in the extremities, the neck (torticollis), and the trunk (pelvic thrust), will accompany the orofacial movement disorder, and occasionally extremity dyskinesia will occur in the absence of orofacial signs. This latter form of the disorder is particularly common in children. Infrequently, the diaphragm and gastrointestinal musculature will be affected, in which case the movement disorder may be life-threatening. A related disorder is Gilles de la Tourette's syndrome, characterized by involuntary movements that are

1

more likely to occur as tics and involuntary vocalizations, of which the most striking and familiar type is coprolalia, but also may include grunting, barking, and jargon (see Chapter 10). Recent case reports suggest that a condition resembling Tourette's syndrome can be induced by chronic neuroleptic treatment.

The etiology of tardive dyskinesia is clearly related to chronic use of agents that block dopamine receptors in the striatum. Thus, antipsychotic (neuroleptic) drugs are most often implicated as the causative agents. The incidence and prevalence of tardive dyskinesia in patients chronically treated with neuroleptic drugs may vary from a few percent to more than 50%, depending on the population studied. Although tardive dyskinesia may be reversible after neuroleptic drugs are discontinued, the symptoms are persistent for many patients and may be disabling. These patients have difficulty in chewing and swallowing, as well as in performing routine daily activities, while the disfigurement of persistent involuntary movements also is socially disabling.

The iatrogenic nature of tardive dyskinesia creates a moral imperative for the physician who prescribes neuroleptic drugs (see Chapter 15). Any iatrogenic disorder is troublesome for the physician as well as for the patient, but the fact that tardive dyskinesia is presently untreatable compounds the problem. It is much easier to accept a disease that occurs naturally, even if it is untreatable, and similarly, an iatrogenic disease for which there is effective treatment is more acceptable. That there is no safe and effective treatment for tardive dyskinesia at this time requires that efforts at prevention of tardive dyskinesia be foremost in the minds of physicians who treat patients at risk (see Chapter 14). All patients receiving neuroleptic drugs have some degree of risk for this complication of neuroleptic therapy, while the highest risk appears to be in the elderly woman who has received neuroleptic therapy for many years and at high doses. However, this does not mean the disorder will not occur in younger patients, or in males, or in those receiving low dose therapy of short duration. Although all neuroleptic drugs have dopamine receptor blockade as their primary pharmacologic action, it appears that receptor blockade in the corpus striatum specifically predisposes to tardive dyskinesia. Therefore, those drugs, which have a high affinity for striatal dopamine receptors, may have a higher likelihood of inducing dyskinesia (see Chapters 11 and 14). Because the typical acute extrapyramidal side effects (EPS) of neuroleptic drugs (parkinsonism) are a direct consequence of striatal dopamine receptor blockade, it is also likely that the propensity of a drug to induce dyskinesia may be related to its propensity to induce acute EPS.

The syndrome of tardive dyskinesia may be progressive while the patient continues to take neuroleptic drugs, but will remain stable, or even improve, after neuroleptic drugs are discontinued. Therefore, it is very important that all patients with signs of tardive dyskinesia be given a trial without neuroleptics. If the patient is able to tolerate withdrawal of neuroleptics, which should be done gradually rather than abruptly, then the chance for improvement of the movement disorder is good. This is especially true when the interval between onset of movement disorder and discontinuation of neuroleptics is very short, whereas those patients who have had dyskinesia for six months or more prior to reduction or discontinuation of neuroleptics are more likely to have a persistent dyskinesia, while it is unlikely the disorder will progress without further exposure to neuroleptics. This contrasts with Huntington's disease, which is inherited as an autosomal dominant gene, and is always progressive. There is no effective treatment for this disorder, although the neuroleptic drugs, particularly haloperidol, are frequently used to control advanced cases in which behavioral and movement symptoms are severely disabling. There is no way to prevent Huntington's disease except by eliminating the gene from the population. The children of an affected parent have a 50% chance of developing the disorder and, once affected, there is no chance for recovery. It is very important to keep in mind the differences between Huntington's disease and tardive dyskinesia (Table 1-1).

The management of a patient with tardive dyskinesia should include discontinuation of neuroleptics and alternative forms of therapy wherever possible (see Chapter 8). For those patients who require continued antipsychotic therapy, careful assessment of the movement disorder should be made periodically, while using the lowest effective dose for the shortest necessary period of time to reduce the long-term risk of worsening the movement disorder. For those patients who require antipsychotic drug therapy and who do not have dyskinesia, using the lowest dose for the shortest period of time, with periodic assessment for the emergence of involuntary movements, will help to reduce the risk. Physicians could dramatically reduce the incidence of tardive dyskinesia by prescribing neuroleptic drugs only on proper indications — generally for psychotic disorders (Chapter 6).

Although no safe and effective treatment for tardive dyskinesia is presently available, research in pursuit of treatments is very active (see Chapters 8, 12, and 13), and there is a possibility that treatment for this condition may be available soon. Another active effort is the search for nonneuroleptic antipsychotic drugs; that is, drugs which have antipsychotic properties without causing neurologic side effects. One such agent, which has been withdrawn from general use due to lethal bone marrow suppression, is clozapine. In extensive European trials, this drug appeared to be a potent antipsychotic, but did not produce EPS.

Table 1-1

	Huntington's Disease	Tardive Dyskinesia
clinical signs	choreiform involuntary movements	
etiology	inherited as autosomal dominant	drug induced
onset	usually late 20's to mid-30's	usually following two or more years of chronic neuroleptic therapy commonly after reduction of dose or discontinuation of neuroleptic
course	always progressive	may be progressive with continued exposure to neuroleptic drugs
	patients usually become severely disabled and die within 10–15 years of onset	will stabilize or improve if neuroleptics can be discontinued
reversibility	none, despite any treatment efforts	yes, in many cases, if neuroleptics are discontinued early
prevention	only if carriers of the gene do not reproduce	with judicious use of neuroleptic drugs and careful monitoring of patients on maintenance therapy
treatment	none	none
	neuroleptic drugs may help to reduce symptoms in severe cases	neuroleptic drugs should be avoided if possible, to prevent progression

Possibly, other such antipsychotic drugs will be available in the future, thus reducing the risk of tardive dyskinesia for patients requiring antipsychotic therapy (see Chapters 8 and 11).

PATHOPHYSIOLOGY

In 1939, Walter Cannon formulated the following *Law of Denervation:*

> When in a series of efferent neurons a unit is destroyed, an increased irritability to chemical agents develops in the isolated structure or structures, the effects being maximal in the part directly denervated.[1]

This hypothesis was the result of observations by Cannon and others that surgical destruction of the presynaptic neuron resulted in hypersensitivity of the postsynaptic neuron to its neurotransmitter. Nearly 30 years later, Carlsson[2] and Klawans,[3] observing that patients with neuroleptic-induced tardive dyskinesia appeared, clinically, to be reacting as if they had an excess of striatal dopaminergic activity, suggested that the pathophysiology of tardive dyskinesia was denervation hypersensitivity to dopamine. The rationale for this hypothesis was as follows:

1. Denervation hypersensitivity results from destruction of the presynaptic neuron, which deprives the postsynaptic membrane of its transmitter.
2. The pharmacologic action of the neuroleptic drugs is blockade of striatal postsynaptic dopamine receptors, which also deprives the postsynaptic membrane of its transmitter.
3. Patients with levodopa intoxication (which produces dopaminergic overactivity) develop movement disorders which are phenomenologically identical to the tardive dyskinesias.
4. Patients with tardive dyskinesia behave, clinically and pharmacologically, as if they have dopaminergic overactivity in the striatum.
5. Depriving the postsynaptic membrane of its transmitter, either by presynaptic neuronal destruction or by postsynaptic receptor blockade, may produce postsynaptic denervation hypersensitivity.

This postsynaptic hypersensitivity hypothesis is supported by abundant clinical and pharmacological evidence, and is now generally accepted as the pathophysiologic basis not only for neuroleptic-induced disorders such as tardive dyskinesia, but also possibly for idiopathic disorders such as Huntington's disease and Gilles de la Tourette's syndrome (see Chapter 10).

Before discussing further the postsynaptic hypersensitivity hypothesis, it is important to review some of the basic and clinical aspects of nigrostriatal function.

The essential anatomic structures involved in the control of voluntary movement are known collectively as the basal ganglia (see Chapter 2). Among these structures, the substantia nigra and the neostriatum are the most critically involved in movement disorders such as Parkinson's disease, Huntington's disease, and tardive dyskinesia. Figure 1-1 illustrates the functional relationship between the substantia nigra and the striatum. The basic element of this relationship is the nigro-striato-nigral feedback loop, the integrity of which is essential for normal control of motor function.

6

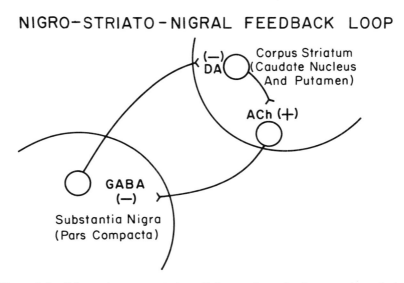

Figure 1-1 Schematic representation of nigro-striato-nigral connections. (−) = inhibitory influence, (+) = facilitatory influence, DA = dopamine, ACh = acetyl choline, GABA = gamma-aminobutyric acid.

This feedback loop consists of a neuron whose cell body originates in the substantia nigra and terminates in the neostriatum (nigrostriatal component), where it releases dopamine (DA), which functions as an inhibitory transmitter for the next neuron in line. This second limb of the loop is an entirely *intra*striatal interneuron, which releases acetyl choline (ACh), and this is a facilitatory transmitter for the next limb of the loop, the striatonigral component. This third neuron has cell body in the neostriatum and terminates in the substantia nigra where it releases gamma-aminobutyric acid (GABA), a transmitter that is inhibitory to the original dopaminergic neuron. Thus, the relationship between these various components of the nigro-striato-nigral feedback loop can be viewed as complementary.

These relationships can also be expressed in terms of the relative balance between dopaminergic and acetyl cholinergic influences in the striatum. This concept of the dopamine-acetyl choline (DA-ACh) balance has gained wide acceptance and, although oversimplifying the situation, facilitates comprehension of the pathophysiologic processes believed to be responsible for movement disorders (Figures 1-2 and 1-3).

The DA-ACh balance hypothesis states there must be a relative balance between these two neurotransmitter systems for normal regulation of voluntary movement to occur. Since the DA system is inhibitory and the ACh system facilitatory (see Figure 1-1), the relationship can be seen as reciprocal. In this reciprocal relationship, reducing dopaminergic

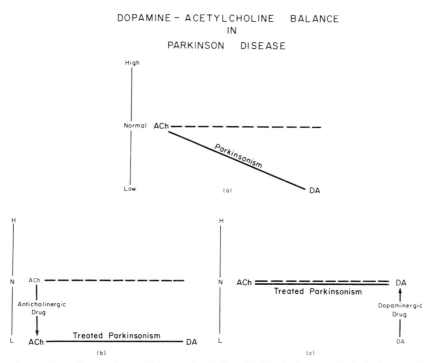

Figure 1-2 Dopamine (DA)-acetyl choline (ACh) balance. **(a)** imbalance of Parkinson's disease and neuroleptic-induced extrapyramidal side-effects (EPS). **(b)** restoration of balance with antiparkinson (anticholinergic) drug treatment. **(c)** restoration of balance with levodopa treatment.

activity or increasing cholinergic activity will result in decreased voluntary movement (hypokinetic movement disorders, ie, Parkinson's disease and neuroleptic-induced EPS), whereas increasing dopaminergic activity or reducing cholinergic activity will result in increased involuntary movements (hyperkinetic movement disorders, ie, Huntington's disease and neuroleptic-induced tardive dyskinesia).

These two types of movement disorders (hypokinetic and hyperkinetic) can now be viewed in terms of both concepts — the nigro-striato-nigral feedback loop and the DA-ACh balance — to clarify both the pathophysiology and the pharmacology of these movement disorders.

Parkinson's Disease and Neuroleptic-induced Extrapyramidal Side-effects (EPS)

The histopathology of idiopathic Parkinson's disease involves degeneration of nigrostriatal dopaminergic neurons, with reduction of

8

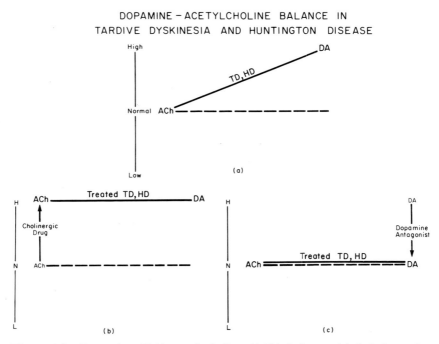

Figure 1-3 Dopamine (DA)-acetyl choline (ACh) balance. **(a)** imbalance in Huntington's disease and neuroleptic-induced tardive dyskinesia. **(b)** restoration of balance with cholinergic drug treatment. **(c)** restoration of balance by dopamine antagonism.

dopaminergic activity in the striatum. The resultant imbalance will be in favor of dopaminergic underactivity and relative cholinergic overactivity (Figure 1-2a), and therapeutic intervention must then be directed at restoring the DA-ACh balance. The most widely used drugs in the treatment of parkinsonism are the anticholinergic (antiparkinson) drugs, and these exert their therapeutic effect by reducing cholinergic activity and restoring the DA-ACh balance (Figure 1-2b). More recently, levodopa, the immediate precursor of dopamine, has been used to treat Parkinson's disease. When given levodopa, patients synthesize excess dopamine, thus making up for the loss of this transmitter due to neuronal degeneration. In this way, levodopa exerts its therapeutic effect by increasing dopaminergic activity to restore the DA-ACh balance (Figure 1-2c).

It is important to note that neuroleptic drug treatment creates the same dopaminergic deficit, albeit by a different mechanism, as that seen in Parkinson's disease. In Parkinson's disease, the mechanism is degeneration of dopaminergic neurons, whereas with neuroleptic drug treatment the mechanism is blockade of postsynaptic striatal dopamine receptors. In either case, the result is reduced dopaminergic activity in the striatum. It is important to note, also, that treatment in either case is accomplished by restoring the DA-ACh balance; indeed, the usual treatment for neuroleptic-induced EPS is with the antiparkinson (anticholinergic) drugs.

Huntington's Disease and Neuroleptic-induced Tardive Dyskinesia

By contrast, Huntington's disease and tardive dyskinesia appear to be clinically and pharmacologically opposite to Parkinson's disease. The histopathology in Huntington's disease involves degeneration of striatal cholinergic and striatonigral gamma-aminobutyric acid releasing (GABAergic) neurons. This results in disinhibition of the nigrostriatal dopaminergic neuron (see Figure 1-1), with the net result of overactivity in the striatal dopaminergic system. Thus, the hyperkinetic movement disorders of Huntington's disease and tardive dyskinesia are characterized by an imbalance favoring dopaminergic overactivity and relative cholinergic underactivity (Figure 1-3a). In this instance, the DA-ACh balance is disturbed in a manner opposite that of Parkinson's disease. Thus, it can be seen that antiparkinson (anticholinergic) drug treatment will actually worsen Huntington's disease and tardive dyskinesia, whereas dopamine antagonism (as with the neuroleptic drugs) will improve or reduce symptoms (Figure 1-3c). Because neuroleptic drug treatment is etiologically implicated in the development of tardive dyskinesia, this treatment, while temporarily relieving symptoms, is not recommended as it recreates the pathogenesis (chronic neuroleptic treatment), and is likely to make tardive dyskinesia worse in the long run. Other approaches to reducing dopaminergic activity as a treatment for tardive dyskinesia are discussed elsewhere in this book (see Chapters 8 and 12). It should be noted, although neuroleptic drugs are not indicated in the treatment of tardive dyskinesia, most experts agree neuroleptic drugs should be used to reduce movement disorder symptoms in patients with Huntington's disease. Whether or not chronic neuroleptic treatment might worsen Huntington's disease is unknown at this time, although the theoretical risk exists. The inevitable progression and relatively short course of Huntington's disease alters the risk/benefit ratio substantially in favor of using neuroleptics in Huntington's disease, as opposed to their use in tardive dyskinesia where the risk may far outweigh the benefit.

On the other side of the DA-ACh balance, if a preponderance of dopaminergic activity is the pathophysiologic basis for tardive dyskinesia, then cholinergic facilitation could restore the balance and be therapeutic for this condition (Figure 1-3b). Drugs known to facilitate cholinergic function, ie, physostigmine, choline, and lecithin (see Chapter 13) have been shown to reduce involuntary movements in some dyskinetic patients, although the long-term risks of such treatment are unknown at this time.

With this background, then, the postsynaptic dopamine hypersensitivity hypothesis can be examined in more detail. The normal dopaminergic system functions basically as illustrated in Figure 1-4a. The presynaptic neuron carries out the synthesis of dopamine from its precursor, dopa. Dopamine is then stored in storage granules, which migrate to the presynaptic cell membrane and release their contents (dopamine) into the synapse, a space which separates the pre- and postsynaptic neurons. On both the pre- and postsynaptic cell membranes are receptor sites to which dopamine binds specifically. This binding can be thought of as a lock and key mechanism, whereby the receptor site recognizes the structural configuration of the correct chemical transmitter (dopamine) and rejects other chemicals. When dopamine is present in the synapse, it will bind to unoccupied dopamine receptors (Figure 1-4b) and neural transmission will occur in the postsynaptic neuron.

The neuroleptic drugs, probably due to some portion of their chemical configuration being similar to that of the dopamine molecule, also have affinity for dopamine receptors, although this is not as strong nor as specific as the affinity of dopamine for the receptor. Thus, these drugs will bind competitively at dopamine receptors and create receptor blockade (Figure 1-5), which prevents dopamine from reaching the receptor site and reduces dopaminergic neural transmission postsynaptically. This is the basis for the neuroleptic-induced EPS, which clinically resemble Parkinson's disease, and which are characterized by striatal (postsynaptic) dopamine deficit (Figure 1-2a). It is presumed that adequate amounts of dopamine are present at the synapse, and normal transmission could occur were it not for the blockade of postsynaptic receptors caused by the presence of the neuroleptic drug. This is confirmed by the fact that patients who develop acute EPS will be restored to normal motor function when neuroleptic drugs are withdrawn.

Now, it may seem paradoxical that drugs known to inhibit dopaminergic activity by blockade of dopamine receptors could ultimately cause the movement disorder of tardive dyskinesia, which is thought to be due to excessive striatal dopaminergic activity. It is important, at this point, to consider the effect which chronic dopamine receptor blockade will have on the postsynaptic neuron, and this is where Cannon's observations on denervation hypersensitivity fit most clearly. Chronic receptor blockade creates a condition in which the postsynaptic membrane is deprived of its neurotransmitter (chemical denervation).

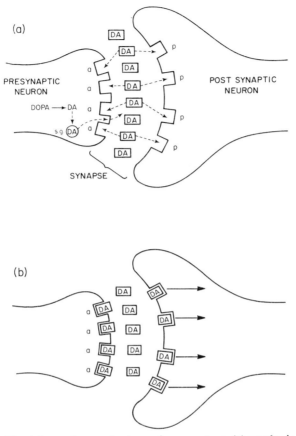

Figure 1-4 Physiology of synaptic dopamine receptors. (a) synthesis and release of dopamine. (b) binding of dopamine at receptor sites. DA = dopamine, sg = storage granule, a = autoreceptor, p = postsynaptic receptor, → = postsynaptic neural transmission.

Thus, the application of Cannon's Law of Denervation suggests the postsynaptic neuron should become hypersensitive. When this hypothesis was first presented to explain tardive dyskinesia more than a decade ago, the mechanism by which this hypersensitivity is produced was unknown. During the last decade, technological developments have permitted the labeling of specific receptors and have resulted in a laboratory procedure that can quantitatively assay dopamine (and other neurotransmitter) receptors. Utilizing this technique, Burt, Creese, and Snyder[4] established that chronic neuroleptic treatment resulted in enhanced dopamine receptor binding, and that this enhancement correlated with behavioral hypersensitivity.[5]

EFFECT OF NEUROLEPTIC DRUGS
(DA RECEPTOR BLOCKADE)

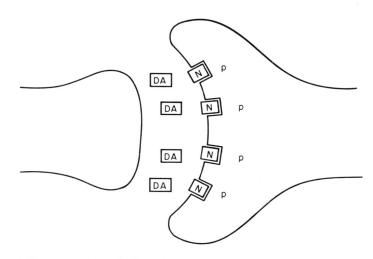

Figure 1-5 Competitive binding of neuroleptic drug (N) to dopamine receptor. DA = dopamine.

This discovery, of the apparent increase in dopamine receptors in response to chronic receptor blockade by neuroleptic drug, represents a significant breakthrough in the study of denervation hypersensitivity, although at the same time it eliminates the apparent paradox mentioned in the preceding paragraph. For what this tells us is that the postsynaptic membrane, faced with the unnatural condition of chronic receptor blockade, follows the fundamental biological principle of homeostasis. Simply stated, this principle requires that any biological system, which is exogenously disrupted (eg, by administration of a drug), will attempt to restore itself, *if possible.* Thus, we would expect the neuroleptically blockaded membrane to attempt to compensate for receptor blockade, and apparently this compensation is accomplished by the *de novo* synthesis of DA receptors (DA receptor hyperplasia) (Figure 1-6a). Thus, with new DA receptors at the postsynaptic membrane, and assuming these are not also blocked by more neuroleptic drug, normal amounts of postsynaptic transmission will occur (Figure 1-6b). This may account for the tolerance to EPS, which is seen in many patients after several weeks of treatment, and also has implications for so-called "breakthrough psychosis" in patients whose psychotic symptoms had been previously adequately controlled.

RESPONSE TO DA RECEPTOR BLOCKADE
(HYPERPLASIA OF RECEPTOR SITES)

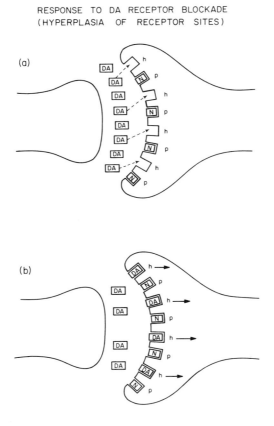

Figure 1-6 **(a)** h = hyperplastic receptor sites synthesized by membrane in response to blockade by neuroleptic drug (N). **(b)** binding of dopamine (DA) to hyperplastic receptor sites (h). → = postsynaptic neural transmission.

The discussion thus far has shown how the postsynaptic membrane compensates for neuroleptic-induced receptor blockade by hyperplasia of receptor sites, which restores the membrane to normal function. This does not, however, explain how hypersensitivity and dopaminergic overactivity are produced. To understand this process, it is necessary to remember that the hyperplasia of receptor sites occurs in the presence of neuroleptic drug, and that some of the DA receptors remain inactivated, or blockaded, by the drug even after new receptors are created (see Figure 1-6b). Thus, while the hyperplastic membrane is *functionally* normal, presumably due to the synthesis of a normal number of *functional* receptor sites, this is not a *physiologically* normal membrane insofar as it

14

has additional *nonfunctional* receptor sites. It is also important to remember that the most common time for the involuntary movements of tardive dyskinesia to appear is after withdrawal of neuroleptic drug, either by reduction of dose or actual discontinuation (see Table 1-1). Withdrawing neuroleptic drug from a hyperplastic membrane will remove the receptor site blockade at some, or all, of the inactivated, or nonfunctional, receptors (Figure 1-7a), thus making them available to bind dopamine and contribute to striatal dopaminergic transmission. The result is a hypersensitive membrane, which will bind excessive amounts of dopamine, resulting in excessive dopaminergic transmission (Figure 1-7b). This excessive dopaminergic transmission manifests clinically as the hyperkinesia of tardive dyskinesia.

EFFECT OF WITHDRAWING NEUROLEPTIC DRUG
FROM HYPERSENSITIVE MEMBRANE

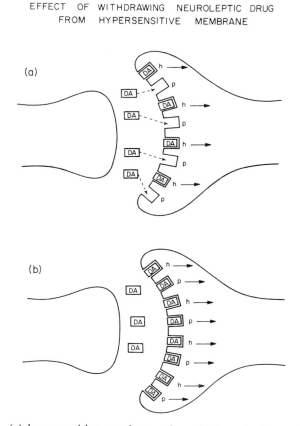

Figure 1-7 **(a)** hypersensitive membrane after withdrawal of neuroleptic drug. Note postsynaptic receptors (p) are free to bind dopamine. **(b)** hypersensitive membrane with additional dopamine (DA) bound to postsynaptic receptor sites. → = postsynaptic neural transmission.

PHARMACOLOGY

The pharmacology of tardive dyskinesia (and Huntington's disease) follows logically, then, from the pathophysiology of these disorders. In a complementary way, the pharmacology of Parkinson's disease, a disorder whose pathophysiology has been described above as being opposite to that of Huntington's disease and tardive dyskinesia, will be opposite as well. In either case, the concepts of the nigro-striato-nigral feedback loop, and the DA-ACh balance, are the basis for nearly all efforts at treatment for these disorders. Various modalities of treatment are discussed in detail in Chapters 8, 12, and 13, and will only be presented here in brief review.

Since the hyperkinetic and hypokinetic movement disorders are not only clinically, but also pathophysiologically, opposite, a generalization can be made about their pharmacology: drugs that improve Parkinson's disease will worsen tardive dyskinesia and Huntington's disease, and vice versa. The pharmacologic actions of the various drugs used in the treatment of these disorders are basically actions that alter the metabolism (either synthesis or degradation) of the neurotransmitters, or that alter receptor-site function (either by agonism or antagonism), and the neurotransmitters and neurotransmitter receptors affected by these drugs will be primarily dopamine, acetyl choline, and gamma-aminobutyric acid.

Parkinson's disease and neuroleptic-induced EPS are treated by reducing cholinergic activity with anticholinergic (antiparkinson) drugs. Levodopa will augment the deficient dopamine system in Parkinson's disease (Figure 1-8), but is not recommended for neuroleptic-induced EPS because of the likelihood of aggravating the underlying psychotic disorder. Dopamine antagonists, such as the neuroleptics, will obviously make Parkinson's disease and EPS worse by further reducing deficient dopaminergic function (see Figure 1-2).

Treatment of Huntington's disease and tardive dyskinesia has focused on all three components of the nigro-striato-nigral feedback loop. The dopaminergic component is overactive in these disorders and treatment efforts are directed at reducing dopaminergic activity via dopamine receptor blockade, depletion of catecholamines, and reducing the synthesis of dopamine (Figure 1-8), or by receptor sensitivity modification (Chapter 12). It should be noted, again, that dopamine receptor blockade by neuroleptic drugs, while reducing symptoms of dyskinesia, may cause long-term aggravation of the disorder, and is not recommended as treatment. Similarly, catecholamine-depleting drugs, ie, reserpine and tetrabenazine, will also reduce symptoms but have been reported to also cause dyskinesia in humans and dopamine receptor hypersensitivity in animals. Obviously, drugs which enhance

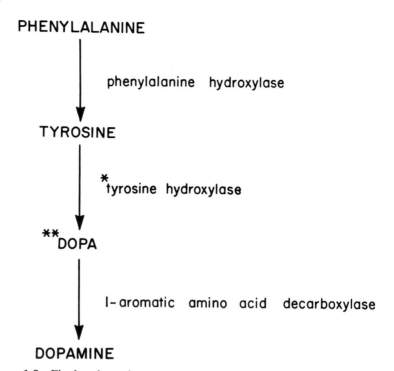

PHENYLALANINE

phenylalanine hydroxylase

TYROSINE

*tyrosine hydroxylase

**DOPA

l-aromatic amino acid decarboxylase

DOPAMINE

Figure 1-8   Final pathway in synthesis of dopamine. *Rate limiting enzyme and point of action for α-methyl-p-tyrosine (tyrosine hydroxylase inhibitor). **Point of action for levodopa in the treatment of Parkinson's disease.

dopaminergic activity will acutely aggravate tardive dyskinesia (see Figure 1-3).

Facilitation of cholinergic function will restore the DA-ACh balance and improve symptoms of tardive dyskinesia, while anticholinergic drugs will aggravate tardive dyskinesia. Acetyl choline synthesis will increase if patients consume large quantities of the precursor, choline or lecithin (Chapter 13). The metabolic degradation of acetyl choline, by acetyl cholinesterase, will be reduced by physostigmine, a cholinesterase inhibitor, thus enhancing cholinergic activity (Figure 1-9).

The GABA system, while probably being the weak link in the feedback system, has been vigorously approached in recent years in efforts to treat tardive dyskinesia and Huntington's disease. Pathologic changes in Huntington's disease involve the degeneration of GABAergic neurons, so augmentation of this system can be viewed as replacement therapy, similar to the use of levodopa in Parkinson's disease. In addition, since the GABAergic neuron is inhibitory on the nigrostriatal dopaminergic neuron (Figure 1-1), it can be seen that facilitating the GABA system will

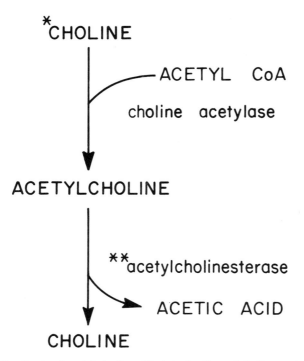

Figure 1-9 Synthesis of acetyl choline. *Point of action of choline and lecithin in the treatment of tardive dyskinesia and Huntington's disease. **Point of action of physostigmine (acetyl cholinesterase inhibitor).

result in reduced striatal dopaminergic activity. Theoretically, GABA synthesis ought to be enhanced by giving large amounts of the precursor, glutamic acid, and possibly by facilitation of the synthetic enzyme, l-aromatic amino acid decarboxylase. Metabolic degradation of GABA can be reduced by inhibiting GABA transaminase, thus enhancing GABAergic transmission (Figure 1-10). Direct-acting GABA receptor agonists will also facilitate GABAergic activity, and recent evidence suggests that the benzodiazepines may stimulate GABAergic neurons.

The pathophysiologic basis for each of the movement disorders discussed above is an imbalance of facilitatory and inhibitory influences in nigrostriatal pathways, and the principle of treatment for these disorders, whether via the DA, ACh, or GABA system, involves restoring the balance of these influences. Thus, although at the present time we have no safe and effective treatment for tardive dyskinesia, our understanding of neurotransmitter function in relation to movement disorders is progressing in a manner that provides a rational foundation for future efforts at treatment.

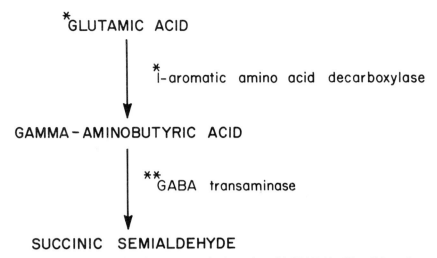

Figure 1-10   Synthesis of gamma-aminobutyric acid (GABA). *Possible points of intervention to increase GABA synthesis. **Point of action of GABA transaminase inhibitors (sodium valproate, gamma-acetylenic-GABA, aminooxyacetic acid).

REFERENCES

1. Cannon WB and Rosenblueth A: *The Supersensitivity of Denervated Structures,* New York, Macmillan, 1949, pp 185–186.
2. Carlsson A: Biochemical implications of dopa-induced actions on the central nervous system, with particular relevance to abnormal movements, in Barbeau A and McDowell FH (eds): *L-Dopa and Parkinsonism.* Philadelphia, Davis, 1970, pp 205–213.
3. Klawans HL: The pharmacology of tardive dyskinesias. *Am J Psychiatry* 130:82–86, 1973.
4. Burt DR, Creese I, and Snyder SH: Antischizophrenic drugs: Chronic treatment elevates dopamine receptor binding in brain. *Science* 196:326–328, 1977.
5. Creese I, Burt DR, and Snyder SH: Dopamine receptor binding enhancement accompanies lesion-induced behavioral supersensitivity. *Science* 197:596–598, 1977.

2 The Anatomy and Physiology of the Basal Ganglia

Richard G. Giaccio

Deep within the brain, in close relationship to the diencephalon but separated from it by the internal capsule, are the large nuclear masses that constitute the basal ganglia. In most common usage, the term basal ganglia is meant to include the caudate nucleus, putamen, and globus pallidus. Some authors still include the claustrum and amygdaloid nuclear complex in the term basal ganglia, although these structures are not functionally related to the first three (Figure 2-1).

Figure 2-2 shows these structures in a schematic form and in selected coronal and horizontal sections. The caudate nucleus is an elongated arched grey mass. Its enlarged anterior portion, or head, bulges into the anterior horn of the lateral ventricle and at this level merges with the putamen laterally. As we proceed posteriorly, the caudate becomes narrowed and is separated from the putamen and globus pallidus by the internal capsule. Further posteriorly, the thalamus appears and becomes increasingly prominent, separated from the lenticular nucleus antero-laterally by the posterior limb of the internal capsule. The body of the

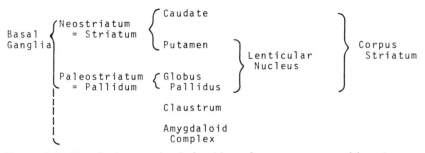

Figure 2-1 Terminology and relationships of structures comprising the extrapyramidal motor system.

caudate lies superolateral to the thalamus and the tail of the caudate finally sweeps into the temporal lobe, lying in the roof of the inferior horn of the lateral ventricle, terminating near the amygdaloid nuclear complex. The putamen and caudate nucleus are phylogenetically the newest part of the basal ganglia, and hence, when taken together are referred to as the new or neostriatum, or, more commonly, simply striatum. They have an identical microscopic appearance and a similar function. The globus pallidus is an older structure and, therefore, is referred to as the paleostriatum or pallidum. It is divided into lateral and medial segments. The putamen and globus pallidus taken together form the lenticular nucleus. While this term has some descriptive use, it adds to the confusion in this area by combining two structures that are anatomically and functionally quite different. The striatum, pallidum, and internal capsule taken collectively are referred to as the corpus striatum. The subthalamic nucleus and the substantia nigra, while not officially included as part of the basal ganglia, are closely related functionally and complete the list of structures comprising the extrapyramidal motor system.

Figure 2-3 shows in block diagram form all of the major structures just discussed and the main fiber pathways connecting them. The striatum can be regarded as the receptive part of the corpus striatum. It receives inputs from nearly all areas of the cerebral cortex, from the intralaminar group of thalamic nuclei, and from the pars compacta of the substantia nigra. Thus, it is the site of conversion for a wide range of inputs. The striatum has a rich neuropil and an abundance of intrinsic neurons, so it is likely that these diverse inputs undergo a considerable degree of integration at this level. The substantia nigra receives its input from the striatum in such a manner that the two are reciprocally and topographically linked, forming a striato-nigro-striatal loop. The major output of the striatum, however, is directed to the pallidum. The pallidum, likewise, has a complex internal structure and maintains a

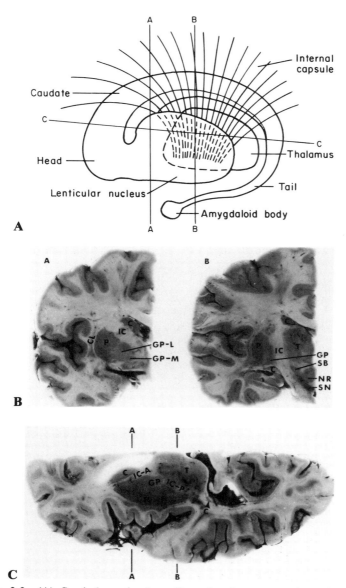

Figure 2-2 **(A)** Semischematic three-dimensional representation of pertinent structures is provided for orientation. **(B)** The level of coronal sections A and B and **(C)** horizontal section C is indicated by vertical lines A and B and horizontal line C respectively. Key: C = Caudate, CL = Claustrum, GP = Globus Pallidus, GP-M = Medial Part, GP-L = Lateral Part, IC = Internal Capsule, IC-A = Anterior Limb, IC-P = Posterior Limb, P = Putamen, SB = Subthalamic Nucleus, NR = Nucleus Ruber, SN = Substantia Nigra, T = Thalamus.

reciprocal relationship with the subthalamic nucleus. The major output of the pallidum projects to parts of the ventral lateral and the ventral anterior thalamic nuclei, which in turn project to the motor (Area 4) and premotor (Area 6) areas of the cerebral cortex. A small part of the pallidal output, however, is directed to the centromedian thalamic nucleus, which may provide some feedback to the striatum (striato-pallido-thalamo-striatal loop), and downward to the midbrain (pedun-culopontine nucleus).

Considering that the basal ganglia are so intimately concerned with motor function, it is very curious that they have no direct access to the lower motor neurons (final common path). Rather, at least by the present state of knowledge, they express themselves solely through their effect upon the motor and premotor areas of the cerebral cortex, and that means ultimately via the direct corticospinal fibers. This, of course, is consistent with the clinical observation that damage to the motor cortex or pyramidal tract abolishes the abnormal involuntary movements (AIM) of extrapyramidal system diseases.

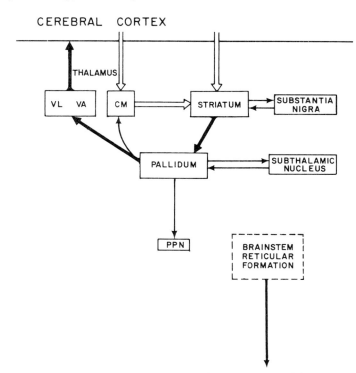

Figure 2-3 Block diagram showing the major structures of the extrapyramidal motor system and their interconnections.

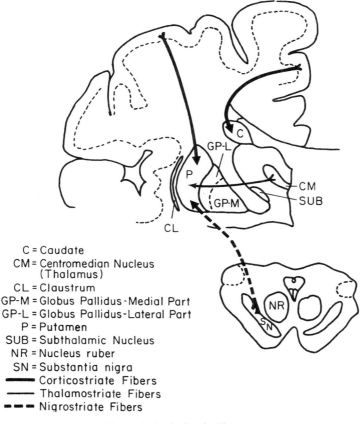

C = Caudate
CM = Centromedian Nucleus
         (Thalamus)
CL = Claustrum
GP-M = Globus Pallidus-Medial Part
GP-L = Globus Pallidus-Lateral Part
P = Putamen
SUB = Subthalamic Nucleus
NR = Nucleus ruber
SN = Substantia nigra
━━ Corticostriate Fibers
─── Thalamostriate Fibers
━ ━ ━ Nigrostriate Fibers

Figure 2-4   Striatal afferents.

Let us now consider each of these pathways in greater detail.

STRIATAL AFFERENTS

As noted above, the striatum receives fibers from the cerebral cortex, the thalamus, and the substantia nigra (see Figure 2-4).

Corticostriate Fibers

Fibers coming from the cerebral cortex are primarily ipsilateral. All regions of the cortex contribute fibers but some areas are more significantly represented. The heaviest projections arise from the somatic sensory and motor areas while association cortex of the frontal and parietotemporal lobes also contributes significantly. These corticostriate fibers are topographically organized in the major dimensions, but there is some overlap of their termination in the striatum. Corticostriate fibers end predominantly upon the dendritic spines of striatal interneurons and are mainly, if not exclusively, excitatory.

Thalamostriate Fibers

The thalamic input to the striatum originates in the intralaminar group of thalamic nuclei. The largest of these, the centromedian (CM) and parafascicular (PF) nuclei, are influenced by fibers from the motor and premotor cortex respectively and project to the putamen. The remaining intralaminar nuclei (mediocentral, paracentral, and lateral-central) receive inputs from ascending sensory tracts, the deep cerebellar nuclei, and the brain stem reticular formation and project primarily to the head of the caudate nucleus. Like the corticostriate fibers, thalamostriate fibers end predominantly upon the dendritic spines of striatal interneurons and are mainly, if not exclusively, excitatory. The transmitter involved in these pathways from the cortex and thalamus is at present unknown, although there is some evidence that it is not acetylcholine.

Nigrostriate Fibers

The substantia nigra has reciprocal and topographically organized connections with the striatum. Nigrostriatal fibers extend from specific regions of the substantia nigra to specific regions of the striatum, and corresponding striatonigral fibers pass in the opposite direction. There is convincing evidence that the nigrostriate fibers are dopaminergic and exert predominantly, although not exclusively, inhibitory effects upon their target cells. Furthermore, histochemical studies have demonstrated that nigrostriatal dopaminergic neurons form direct synapses on cholinergic interneurons of the striatum, thus providing a likely anatomic basis for the dopaminergic-cholinergic link long hypothesized on the basis of clinical and pharmacologic data. There is some evidence that there may be one or more additional fiber tracts running parallel to the dopaminergic nigrostriate fibers but utilizing other neurotransmitters, possibly serotonin or norepinephrine. Going in the opposite direction, recent studies indicate that there are two types of descending striatonigral fibers, one that is inhibitory and uses GABA as its transmitter, the second is excitatory and utilizes the polypeptide substance P. Thus, it appears that the reciprocally related fibers running from the substantia nigra to the striatum and vice versa form a striato-nigral-striatal loop, which probably functions as a neuronal feedback circuit. This loop may function to maintain a certain homeostasis of the dopaminergic influence on the striatum (see Chapter 1).

STRIATAL EFFERENTS – PALLIDAL AFFERENTS

Of all the cells in the striatum, only a very few (perhaps 1 in 20 to 1 in 60) give rise to efferents that leave the nucleus (see Figure 2-5). Some of these fibers, as noted above, pass to the substantia nigra. The bulk of striatal output, however, passes to the globus pallidus. These striatopallidal projections are topographically organized and radiate to

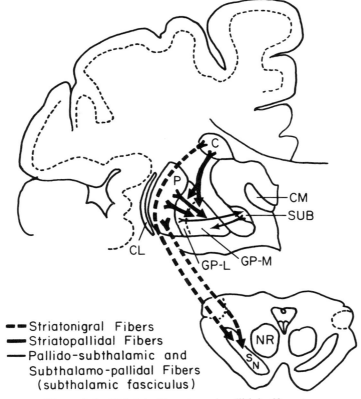

Figure 2-5 Striatal efferents and pallidal afferents.

the pallidum like the spokes of a wheel, giving off collaterals to both pallidal segments. Fibers from the striatum are thought to be primarily inhibitory upon pallidal target cells and utilize GABA as their neurotransmitter. Electrophysiologic studies indicate that the striatopallidal and striatonigral inhibitory fibers are collateral from the same perikaryon. Other studies have shown excitatory as well as inhibitory effects in the pallidum from striatal stimulation. It can only be speculated at this point in time whether this implies a second excitatory striatopallidal pathway parallel to the major inhibitory GABAergic system, or whether this represents the response of different types of pallidal receptors to the same neurotransmitter.

Subthalamic Nucleus

The subthalamic nucleus receives its input from the lateral pallidal segment and sends its output primarily to the medial pallidal segment. Lesions of the subthalamic nucleus result in the violent dyskinesia of hemiballismus and suggest that the fibers originating in the subthalamic nucleus exert an inhibitory influence upon neurons in the medial pallidal segment. There is some suggestion that glycine may be the inhibitory transmitter in this pathway.

PALLIDAL EFFERENTS

Fibers arising from the medial pallidal segment form the principal efferents system of the basal ganglia (Figure 2-6) and are organized into two bundles, the ansa lenticularis and the fasciculus lenticularis (H_2). These bundles follow a distinctive course in relation to the internal capsule but merge in Forel's field H. Fibers then pass rostrally and laterally in the thalamic fasciculus to terminate in parts of the ventral lateral (VL) and ventral anterior (VA) thalamic nuclei. While the bulk of pallidothalamic fibers pass to VL and VA, a few fine fibers separate from the thalamic fasciculus and terminate in the centromedian (CM) thalamic nucleus, thus providing feedback to the striatum. The medial pallidal segment also gives rise to several smaller projections whose functional significance is unclear at this time. These include pallidotegmental fibers terminating in the pedunculopontine nucleus of the caudal midbrain and pallidohabenular fibers terminating in the lateral habenular nucleus. The latter projections suggest a possible relationship of the basal ganglia to the limbic system. The neurotransmitters involved in the pallidofugal system are at present unknown. These fibers are believed to be primarily excitatory upon their thalamic target cell. At this point, it might be mentioned that the substantia nigra also sends some fibers to the VL and VA thalamic nuclei. These fibers appear to be a second pathway from the striatum to the thalamus parallel to the more significant route through the globus pallidus.

THALAMUS

To complete the picture, it should be noted that the ventral lateral and ventral anterior thalamic nuclei project respectively to the motor (Area 4) and premotor (Area 6) areas of cerebral cortex, and that through these connections they can influence the output of the pyramidal neurons that give rise to the corticospinal tracts. Thus it is that the influence of the basal ganglia finally reaches the lower motor neuron and achieves motor expression.

Figure 2-7 summarizes some of the anatomic, electrophysiologic, and neurochemical data that have just been reviewed. It should be emphasized that this is a simplified model and that in reality things are probably much more complex. It shows the excitatory fibers coming into the striatum from the cerebral cortex and thalamus, and the reciprocal relationships of the striatum and the substantia nigra. Inhibitory dopaminergic fibers pass from the nigra to the striatum where they synapse on excitatory cholinergic interneurons, which in turn synapse on

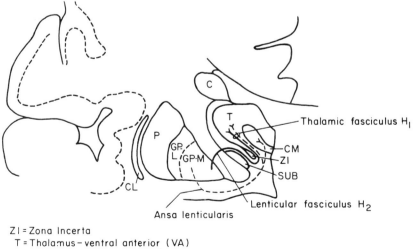

ZI = Zona Incerta
T = Thalamus – ventral anterior (VA)
        ventral lateral (VL)

Figure 2-6 Pallidal efferents.

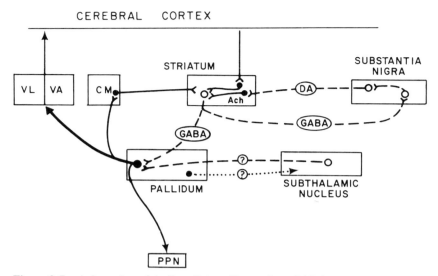

Figure 2-7 Ach = Acetylcholine, DA = Dopamine, GABA = γ-Aminobutyric Acid, Excitatory Fibers ____, Inhibitory Fibers - - - -, Function unknown . . . .

inhibitory GABAergic neurons whose fibers form the striatal efferents. What is depicted here is really the simplest kind of connectivity, and one could imagine that there might well be whole series of interneurons interposed between the striatal inputs and outputs. In any case, inhibitory GABAergic fibers ultimately leave the striatum. Some pass to the substantia nigra to complete that feedback loop and the bulk pass to the pallidum, where, either directly or via internuncials, they influence units giving rise to excitatory pallidal efferents, which in turn pass to the thalamus (the VL and VA) and thence to the cortex.

This model, while certainly oversimplified, has some utility in conceptualizing some of the clinical and pharmacologic data regarding certain basal ganglia disorders. In Parkinson's disease the primary lesion is believed to be a deficiency in nigrostriatal dopamine. A decrease in dopamine release at the synapse in the striatum leads to a decrease in inhibition of a cholinergic interneuron, which then fires at an increased rate and causes increased excitation of the GABAergic neurons. Increased firing of these neurons leads to an increased inhibition of pallidal neurons whose output is normally excitatory upon thalamic, and thence cortical, neurons producing a state of hypokinesia. Conversely, an excess of dopamine, such as might result from toxic doses of levodopa, would have the opposite effect and initiate a sequence resulting in a hyperkinetic state, which is in fact what is observed clinically. It can also be seen from this model how an anticholinergic drug might counteract the effect of dopamine deficiency. The model is consistent with the finding of decreased GABA in the caudate of patients suffering from Huntington's disease. In this case the loss of GABAergic fibers would lead to insufficient inhibition of the pallidal neurons and hence a hyperkinetic state.

At this point, it may be worth reviewing briefly some of the proposals that have been made concerning the function of the basal ganglia in the intact organism. One theory proposed by Wilson in 1928 is that the primary function of the basal ganglia is to maintain a postural background for voluntary activities, reinforcing and steadying movements, and postures of cortical origin, but incapable of initiating such movements. Thus, in a certain sense, the basal ganglia could be seen as a higher level system whose function is nonetheless kin to that of the vestibulospinal and reticulospinal systems. While it is true that people with basal ganglia disease often show marked abnormalities in posture, the symptomatology is of course much richer. There is the akinesia and tremor of parkinsonism, the hyperkinesia of Huntington's disease, etc. There is also the observation that in submammalian vertebrates and even in cats, a whole range of complex behaviors including locomotion, defense, feeding, and courting are integrated at the level of the basal ganglia, and that extirpation of the primitive cerebral cortex causes little or no interference with these functions. These data suggest a more complex role for the basal ganglia.

Some authors have proposed that the basal ganglia contain preprogrammed neural circuits for the control of stereotyped behavioral sequences. Another way of stating this idea would be that rather than having to have the cortex generate commands for the exact timing and sequence of individual muscle contraction every time it wants to initiate an activity, rather than going through all of that, brief sequences of motor activity are preprogrammed or hardwired into the basal ganglia. The cortex simply activates these preprogrammed neural circuits in the appropriate order to produce the desired behavior. Hypokinesia would represent the loss or inability to activate these circuits. Hyperkinesia would be seen as the disinhibition or discontrol (release) of these neuromechanisms. Observation of patients with chorea tends to support this view. It has long been commented that their abnormal involuntary movements resemble brief snatches of normal motor activity and that these patients frequently try to *cover up* these abnormal movements by making them flow into some completed and seemingly purposeful action. The wiring pattern discussed previously is consistent with this. The basal ganglia, after sampling diverse regions of the cerebral cortex, process the data and then project to circumscribed areas of the cortex, that is, the motor and premotor areas. Several authors have called atten-

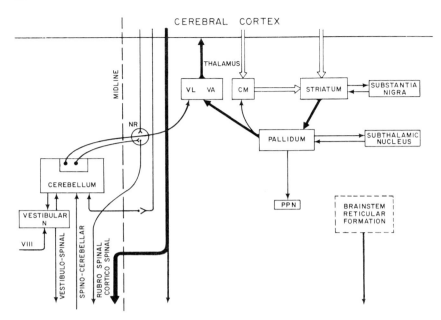

Figure 2-8 Block diagram showing the relationship of the extrapyramidal, cerebellar, and corticospinal motor systems.

tion to the similarities between the extrapyramidal system and the cerebellar system (Figure 2-8).

Like the basal ganglia, the cerebellum receives input from diffuse areas of cerebral cortex, integrates this with other inputs and then projects via thalamic relays to circumscribed areas of the cerebral cortex, specifically Area 4. Thus, the extrapyramidal and cerebellar systems are connected in parallel between diffuse cortical areas and other inputs on one hand, and specific cortical motor areas on the other. Some authors have suggested that the basal ganglia function primarily in the generation of slow (ramp) movements, whereas the cerebellum functions largely in the preprogramming and initiation of rapid (saccadic) movements, which do not make use of sensory feedback. This theory differs considerably from the classic notion of the cerebellar system functioning as a servo-mechanism for the *fine tuning* or coordination of movements on the basis of peripheral proprioceptive feedback.

It is of particular interest that cerebellar efferents project to the ventral lateral thalamic nucleus, which also receives efferents from the basal ganglia. Some believe that there is a considerable overlap of these projections in VL, and that some degree of integration of cerebellar and basal ganglia output is taking place at this level. Others maintain that cerebellar and basal ganglia fibers project to different portions of VL and that there is little overlap or integration, and that whereas the cerebellar output is relayed to the motor cortex (Area 4), the pallidal output, even that going through VL and all of that going through VA, actually projects diffusely to the frontal lobe.

Finally, while there can be no doubt as to the importance of the basal ganglia in somatic motor function, there is a growing body of evidence that disorders of basal ganglia produce more than purely motor deficits. For example, on certain tasks of spatial orientation (body scheme and route walking), parkinsonian patients made significantly more errors than controls matched for age and verbal IQ. Other studies have shown defects in concept formation, shifting of sets, and in short-term memory of visual, auditory, and kinestatic material. These defects occur in the absence of general intellectual deterioration or primary deficits in the registration of sensory stimuli, and do not correlate with the degree of tremor, rigidity, or akinesia.

In summary, an attempt has been made to define the basic structures comprising the extrapyramidal motor system, to review their major connections with each other and with various parts of the CNS and to fill in the bones of this skeleton with what is known of the actions of the various fibers, the terms of excitation and inhibition, and the neurotransmitters they employ. A simplified model was presented synthesizing much of the above data. In closing, some speculations have been made as to the role of the basal ganglia in overall motor function and its relationship to the cerebellar and corticospinal systems; and finally some evidence has been offered, which suggests a role of the basal ganglia in certain perceptual and cognitive functions.

BIBLIOGRAPHY

Baldessarini RJ, Tarsy P: Mechanisms underlying tardive dyskinesia, in Yahr MD (ed): *The Basal Ganglia*. New York, Raven Press, 1976.

Bowen FP: Behavioral alterations in patients with basal ganglia lesions, in Yahr MD (ed.): *The Basal Ganglia*. New York, Raven Press, 1976.

Carlsson A: Some aspects of dopamine in the basal ganglia, in Yahr MD (ed): *The Basal Ganglia*. New York, Raven Press, 1976.

Carpenter MB: Anatomical organization of the corpus striatum and related nuclei, in Yahr MD (ed): *The Basal Ganglia*. New York, Raven Press, 1976.

Chase TN: Serotonergic mechanisms and extrapyramidal function in man, in McDowell FH, Barbeau A (eds): *Advances in Neurology,* vol 5. New York, Raven Press, 1974.

DeLong MR: Activity of pallidal neurons during movement. *J Neurophysiol* 34:414, 1971.

DeLong MR: Motor functions of the basal ganglia: Single-unit activity during movement, in Schmitt FO, Worden FG (eds): *Neurosciences: Third Study Program.* Cambridge, MIT Press, 1974, pp 319–325.

DeLong MR, Strick PL: Relation of basal ganglion, cerebellum, and motor cortex units to ramp and ballistic limb movements. *Brain Res* 71:327–335, 1974.

Denny-Brown D, Yanagisawa N: The role of the basal ganglia in the initiation of movement, in Yahr MD (ed): *The Basal Ganglia*. New York, Raven Press, 1976.

Fahn S: Biochemistry of the basal ganglia, in Eldridge R, Fahn S (eds): *Advances in Neurology,* vol 14. New York, Raven Press, 1976.

Gale K, Hong J-S, Guidotti A: Presence of substance P and GABA in separate striatonigral neurons. *Brain Res* 136:371–375, 1977.

Guyton AC: Chaps 52 and 53, in *Textbook of Medical Physiology,* ed 5. Philadelphia, W.B. Saunders, 1976, pp 694–708; 710–727.

Teuber H-L: Complex functions of basal ganglia, in Yahr MD (ed): *The Basal Ganglia*. New York, Raven Press, 1976.

Nauta HJW: Evidence of a pallidohabenular pathway in the cat. *J Comp Neuro* 156:19–28, 1974.

Kemp JM, Powell TPS: The termination of fibres from the cerebral cortex and thalamus upon dendritic spines in the caudate nucleus: A study with the Golgi method. *Philos Trans R Soc Lond (Biol)* 262:429–439, 1971.

Kemp JM, Powell TPS: The structure of the caudate nucleus of the cat: Light and electron microscopy. *Philos Trans R Soc Lond (Biol)* 262:383–401, 1971.

Kemp JM, Powell TPS: The synaptic organization of the caudate nucleus. *Philos Trans R Soc Lond (Biol)* 262:403–412, 1971.

Kemp JM, Powell TPS: The site of termination of afferent fibres in the caudate nucleus. *Philos Trans R Soc Lond (Biol)* 262:413–427, 1971.

Kemp JM, Powell TPS: The connexions of the striatum and globus pallidus: Synthesis and speculation. *Philos Trans R Soc Lond (Biol)* 262:441–457, 1971.

Klawans HL: The pharmacology of extrapyramidal movement disorders, in *Monographs in Neural Sciences,* vol 2. Basel, Karger, 1973.

Kornhuber HH: Cerebral cortex, cerebellum and basal ganglia: An introduction to their motor functions, in Schmitt FO, Worden FG (eds): *Neurosciences: Third Study Program*. Cambridge, MIT Press, 1974, pp 267–280.

McGeer PL, Hatton T, Singh VK, et al: Cholinergic systems in extrapyramidal function, in Yahr MD (ed): *The Basal Ganglia*. New York, Raven Press, 1976.

McLennan H, York PH: The action of dopamine on neurones of the caudate nucleus. *J Physiol* 189:393–402, 1967.

Okada Y, Nitsch-Hassler C, Kim JS, et al: Role of aminobutyric acid (GABA) in the extrapyramidal motor system. *Exp Brain Res* 13:514–518, 1971.

Poirier LN, Parent A, Roberge AG: The striatopallidal system: Its implication in motor disorders. *Pathobiol Annu* 5:339–367, 1975.

Purpura DP: Physiologic organization of the basal ganglia, in Yahr MD (ed): *The Basal Ganglia*. New York, Raven Press, 1976.

Roberts E: Some thoughts about GABA and the basal ganglia, in Yahr MD (ed): *The Basal Ganglia*. New York, Raven Press, 1976.

3 Epidemiology of Tardive Dyskinesia: Part 1

Joseph DeVeaugh-Geiss

The reported prevalence rates for tardive dyskinesia show considerable variation, with one older study reporting 0.5%,[1] and more recent studies reporting greater than 40%[2-6] of patients developing tardive dyskinesia. The very recent literature shows about a 30% to 50% prevalence rate in inpatients as well as outpatients, suggesting that the magnitude of the problem is greater than previously had been realized.

Tardive dyskinesia recently has assumed another kind of significance, in addition to its clinical significance, and this has to do with medical malpractice. Decisions regarding the requirement to disclose a risk, held up as standards in malpractice litigation, suggest that any severe complication of treatment, which appears in 3% of patients receiving the treatment, will be considered to be a significant risk and the courts will recognize this degree of risk as cause for disclosure[7] (see also, Chapter 15). The literature does not specify whether the frequency of occurrence referred to here is incidence or prevalence, but if a complication appears with a frequency of 3% it should be disclosed, which means simply the patient should be advised that the particular risk may accompany the treatment. Regardless of the legal issues, 50%, 30%, and even 25% prevalence is a very high rate of complication and probably would not be acceptable for most therapies in other disciplines of medicine. Jus, in 1976,[8] studied a large population of chronically hospitalized patients, separated his patient population by age, and found that those under the age of 49 showed a 40% prevalence, those between the ages of 50 and 70 showed a 60% prevalence, and those above the age of 70 showed a 75% prevalence of tardive dyskinesia. Other studies support this finding, suggesting that it would be well to follow the advice given by Doctor Crane regarding conservative use of neuroleptics in elderly patients who appear to be at very high risk for dyskinesia.[9]

Another aspect of the epidemiology of tardive dyskinesia, especially regarding risk factors, is the very confusing literature. Nearly everything that has been reported is contradicted in another report. Correlations found in one study are not found in other studies. Although there are replications, or several reports of the same findings, there are frequently as many reports of the contrary finding. It is unknown how the various investigators decided which factors they would study in association with tardive dyskinesia, but some of the factors that have been commonly studied are: previous brain damage, previous electric shock treatment, the sex of the patient, the length of hospitalization, the duration and dose of neuroleptic treatment, and the nature of the patient's response to treatment. In all of the reported studies, some of these factors are correlated with dyskinesia and others are not, but there is little correlation of the findings between studies, and there does not seem to be any compelling evidence to support a judgment at this time about many of these factors necessarily predisposing to tardive dyskinesia.

A different approach, which has been used more recently, involves examining specific aspects of these potential risk factors. For example, the one factor that is highly correlated with tardive dyskinesia is age, and in all studies the prevalence figures are always highest in the oldest patient populations. Some studies have looked further into that finding and, for example, have tried to determine whether age at the time of initiation of treatment is a significant factor as this might correspond to duration of treatment. After all, if consistent results are not found regarding duration of treatment, the age at onset of treatment might be found to be a differentiating feature. One survey asked that question, and found there was a higher incidence of dyskinesia in people who were older when they started their treatment, even if they were treated for the same duration and with roughly equivalent drug dosages.[8]

Others have looked at the question of drug dosage from another perspective. Perhaps, certain types of drugs in the same or equivalent doses have more or less propensity to induce dyskinesias. Although this question certainly is open, there have been some reports that implicate treatment with fluphenazine (Prolixin) more highly as a risk factor in tardive dyskinesia,[10-12] and in one of these reports there was negative correlation with thioridazine (Mellaril) treatment.[12] Whether those factors will be consistently found in subsequent studies remains to be seen, but looking at more detailed aspects of risk factors might help to clarify the inconsistencies (see also Chapters 11 and 14).

The question about sex or gender of the patient also shows conflicting results. Some studies have found dyskinesia to be more prevalent in females than in males,[2,4,13,14] while others have found the male/female difference in prevalence to be insignificant.[6,15,16] This does not really tell much, although one study looked at this question in more detail and found a correlation between sex and age, so that if populations are examined over a broad range of age, very little in the way of sex differences in the younger populations is found, with males and females being more or less equally affected, while with older age groups, a significant increase is found in the prevalence of tardive dyskinesia among the female patients.[17] Thus, studies that concentrate on younger patients will necessarily find a different kind of sex difference than those that focus only on the elderly patients. This kind of information is beginning to elucidate some of the very fine points that may be responsible for the very confusing literature.

One of the recent studies, which implicates fluphenazine more often than other neuroleptics in the development of tardive dyskinesia, found a 31% prevalence rate in an outpatient population.[11] These investigators also found, as most have, an increase in tardive dyskinesia among patients who are older. Interestingly, they also found that the duration of hospitalization seems to correlate with the prevalence of tardive dyskinesia. This is a curious finding, because it does not correspond to duration of neuroleptic drug treatment, but only to duration of hospitalization. Early studies reported that previous brain damage and previous electroconvulsive treatments increased the risk for dyskinesias, while subsequent reports did not find that correlation. In this study, however, a correspondence was found between the existence of organic brain syndrome and the severity of the dyskinesia. This finding fits well with data from my own patient population, in which the more severe movement disorders were found in patients with preexisting brain damage, whereas the milder disorders were seen in patients who showed no evidence of brain damage. In the study mentioned above by Chouinard et al, the more severe disorders were also found more often among the male patients, so it appears that studies utilizing very stringent criteria and only including the severe movement disorders will probably find a different rate of prevalence among males and females than will studies which include the milder dyskinesias.

This suggests that perhaps the detection of the disorder—the actual diagnosis or methodology employed in these studies—could be responsible for the equivocal findings. What one person calls dyskinesia may not be what another calls dyskinesia. There was an argument about the correct diagnosis in a sample of patients who were reported in a preliminary drug trial to have responded to lecithin. A knowledgeable and respected investigator wrote to the journal that published the report and said that he had seen movies of the patients from that study, and they appeared to him to have parkinsonian tremor and dystonia rather than tardive dyskinesia.[18]

There are very few objective criteria for assessment of tardive dyskinesia. The National Institute of Mental Health has developed a standard examination procedure and rating scale, the abnormal involuntary movement scale, or AIMS[19] (see Appendix 2). But, even when using this scale there are various cut-off criteria that could be used along the scale to determine whether a patient has or does not have tardive dyskinesia. So, imagine that perhaps the more severe disorders are more common in people with organic brain syndromes and the investigators are only diagnosing tardive dyskinesia when it is very severe. Such a study will find a very biased prevalence figure that will point to a correlation between organic brain syndrome and tardive dyskinesia; this could occur similarly in evaluating sex differences.

Another important methodological problem, which complicates understanding the epidemiology of tardive dyskinesia, is that virtually all the data on hand is retrospective. Someone will take a sample of patients with the diagnosis of tardive dyskinesia, and review their records and make comparisons. There is some value in this method as it may lead to particular areas of inquiry that might be fruitful, but valid judgments about etiologies, risk factors, and cause/effect relationships cannot be made from retrospective studies. In fact, this frequently cannot be done with longitudinal, or prospective, studies; the type of study that begins today with a cohort and follows patients over a period of time, makes periodic assessments at arbitrary time intervals, and then determines an incidence rate for a certain disorder. But such an approach is more valid because it is less biased. There appears to have been only one longitudinal study of tardive dyskinesia.[20] It involved a large number of patients, and observations were made of motor side effects from neuroleptic treatment while the patients were treated as they normally would be in the hospital. The study itself was not designed to modify the patients' treatment, although some patients were withdrawn from neuroleptics and others had certain other modifications imposed on their drug treatment.

The results of this study revealed that patients who had no dyskinesia when they entered the study showed about a 50% rate of dyskinesia after one year. This suggests an incidence of 50% and is the only incidence figure currently available. Probably the most interesting finding from this study is that the people who entered the study with dyskinesia showed a reduction of symptoms after one year. When the study group was broken down according to medication status, the frequency of dyskinesia correlated with whether or not the patients were withdrawn or maintained under neuroleptic treatment. Those without dyskinesia who were maintained during one year showed a high incidence of dyskinesia at the end of that time, and those who started with dyskinesia and were maintained may have still had dyskinesia after one year, but many of those dyskinetic patients who were withdrawn from neuroleptics showed a loss of their dyskinetic symptoms at one-year follow up. This suggests the advice that has been heard and given for years now, that at early signs of dyskinesia, neuroleptic medication should be discontinued, is good advice and perhaps it can be expected that over a period of time some patients with tardive dyskinesia will get better after withdrawal of neuroleptic medication.

It is unfortunate more studies of this type have not been done, but this is a very cumbersome and difficult procedure to follow. Another finding in this study was a high degree of correlation between the development of extrapyramidal side effects during treatment with neuroleptics and subsequent development of dyskinesia. This is where Crane first reported the transition from parkinsonian side effects to the more hyperkinetic, dyskinetic phenomena described as tardive dyskinesia. That is very important and corresponds to other reports, although there is equivocation in the literature on this point as well. Some reports have suggested that previous antiparkinsonian (anticholinergic) drug treatment may increase the risk for tardive dyskinesia,[21] while others have not found that to be the case.[8,11] Among the people studied by me, previous antiparkinsonian drug treatment was found to be a common part of the history, but usually because the people had extrapyramidal side effects that were being treated. There have been a few patients who did not receive antiparkinsonian drug treatment but nevertheless had extrapyramidal side effects (EPS) that were very detectable and obvious. These patients had untreated EPS for some time and then ultimately progressed to a dyskinesia. It is my opinion that the EPS, not the antiparkinsonian drug, may be the significant factor.

In my own study, which included detailed information for 30 people with tardive dyskinesia who have been seen very recently, something was found that is being reported by others: a higher frequency either of depressive symptoms in the population of dyskinetic patients, regardless of diagnosis, or a higher risk for tardive dyskinesia associated with the existence of an affective type of disorder previously.[22,23] In this group, 13 were diagnosed as schizophrenic, while nine were treated with neuroleptics for depression. Although some of those had what was described as psychotic depression, 9 of 30 is a large number of people with a diagnosis of depression and receiving neuroleptic treatment, which usually is reserved for different kinds of disorders. It is uncertain whether that is a sampling bias because only people who had dyskinesia were selected or whether it generally might be true that a large number of depressed people are being treated with neuroleptic drugs.

In my patient population, it has been consistently found that the reversibility of dyskinesia (a very important clinical issue) seems to correspond to two things; the main one being the duration of the dyskinesia following its appearance before neuroleptics have been discontinued. In 10 of these 30 patients, the dyskinesia was reversible, and in all ten of these, the initial appearance of the dyskinesia and the subsequent withdrawal of neuroleptics occurred within six months, whereas the irreversible dyskinesias were present longer than six months before any change of neuroleptic drug occurred. A correspondence between the existence of previous brain damage and reversibility was seen, with brain damaged patients having more irreversible dyskinesias. Reversibility is, of course, a crucial factor. If tardive dyskinesia can be prevented, that is fine. If it cannot be prevented and patients develop dyskinesia, everything should be done to make it reversible because it cannot be treated.

An observation about extrapyramidal side effects should be mentioned. Tardive dyskinesia can be thought of as an extrapyramidal phenomenon, and not very different from acute extrapyramidal side effects, ie, tremor, pseudoparkinsonism, and dystonia. It is a variant of these and behaves differently pharmacologically. Some people who have been followed over a long period of time, from initiation of the neuroleptic treatment until the development of their dyskinesia, have shown the progression of symptoms described by Crane (see Chapter 14). One of these people developed a very rigid and hyperkinetic extrapyramidal syndrome, which began with some rigidity, some jerky movements in ambulation (he looked like he was marching rather than walking) that were associated with akathisia. This syndrome persisted for roughly one week, until the involuntary tongue movements appeared.

Interestingly, it appears that this man, although he had the lingual involuntary movements, responded pharmacologically as if he had a pseudoparkinsonian reaction; ie, the lingual movements diminished when the patient was given the anticholinergic drug, benztropine, and they rapidly disappeared when neuroleptics were withdrawn. Another patient presented a similar movement disorder, sort of a *marching* syndrome with rigidity and tremor, but with a very marked hyperkinetic tremor and akathisia that immediately preceded by a week or ten days the onset of the orofacial dyskinesia. In both of these cases, the dyskinesia was fully and promptly reversible upon discontinuation of neuroleptics and did not worsen when neuroleptics were withdrawn, as usually is seen in people with late-appearing dyskinesia. These two patients may have had an extrapyramidal reaction which represented a transitional phase between acute, drug-induced parkinsonism and tardive dyskinesia, and this syndrome, if allowed to progress, ie, if neuroleptic drugs were continued, could have become a classic tardive dyskinesia (see also Chapter 8, *Differential Diagnosis*).

In summary, little information is available at this time regarding predictors or risk factors, although the evidence is compelling that age is a risk factor. It is not a predictor, but advanced age increases the risk for tardive dyskinesia. It is also likely that the appearance of extrapyramidal phenomena in a patient may signal a sensitivity in that part of the nervous system that controls voluntary movement, and that this may predispose the patient to the subsequent development of dyskinetic phenomena.

REFERENCES

1. Hoff H, Hoffman G: Das persistierende extrapyramidale syndrom bei neuroleptika therapie. *Wien Med Wochenschr* 117:14–17, 1967.

2. Kennedy PF, Hershon HI, McGuire LH: Extrapyramidal disorders after prolonged phenothiazine therapy. *Br J Psychiatry* 118:509–518, 1971.

3. Smith JM, Oswald WT, Kucharski LT, et al: Tardive dyskinesia: Age and sex differences in hospitalized schizophrenics. *Psychopharmacol* 58:207–211, 1978.

4. Bell RCH, Smith RC: Tardive dyskinesia: Characterization and prevalence in a statewide system. *J Clin Psychiatry* 39:39–42, 1978.

5. Jus A, Pineau R, LaChance R, et al: Epidemiology of tardive dyskinesia: Part I. *Dis Nerv Syst* 37:210–214, 1976.

6. Asnis GM, Leopold MA, Duvoisin RC, et al: A survey of tardive dyskinesia in psychiatric outpatients. *Am J Psychiatry* 134:1367–1370, 1977.

7. Louisell DW, Williams H: *Medical Malpractice,* vol 2. New York, Matthew Bender, 1975, p 594.47.

8. Jus A, Pineau R, LaChance R, et al: Epidemiology of tardive dyskinesia: Part II. *Dis Nerv Syst* 37:257–261, 1976.

9. Crane GE: The prevention of tardive dyskinesia. *Am J Psychiatry* 134:756–758, 1977.

10. Gardos G, Cole JO, LaBrie RA: Drug variables in the etiology of tardive dyskinesia-discriminant function analysis. *Prog Neuropsychopharm* 1:147–154, 1977.

11. Chouinard G, Annable L, Ross-Chouinard A, et al: Factors related to tardive dyskinesia. *Am J Psychiatry* 136:79–83, 1979.

12. Smith RC, Strizich M, Klass M: Drug history and tardive dyskinesia. *Am J Psychiatry* 135:1402–1403, 1978.

13. Smith JM, Kucharski LT, Oswald WT, et al: A systematic investigation of tardive dyskinesia in inpatients. *Am J Psychiatry* 136:918–922, 1979.

14. Brandon S, McClelland HA, Protheroe C: A study of facial dyskinesia in a mental hospital population. *Br J Psychiatry* 118:171–184, 1971.

15. Fann WE, Davis JM, Janowsky DS: The prevalence of tardive dyskinesias in mental hospital patients. *Dis Nerv Syst* 33:182–186, 1972.

16. Crane GE, Paulson G: Involuntary movements in a sample of chronic mental patients and their relation to the treatment with neuroleptics. *Int J Neuropsychiatry* 3:286–291, 1966.

17. Smith JM, Dunn DD: Sex differences in the prevalence of severe tardive dyskinesia. *Am J Psychiatry* 136:1080–1082, 1979.

18. Fahn S: Tardive dyskinesia may be only akathisia. *N Engl J Med* 299:202–203, 1978.

19. Guy W: *ECDEU Assessment Manual for Psychopharmacology.* US Department of Health, Education and Welfare, Psychopharmacology Research Branch, DHEW Publication #76-338, 1976, pp 534–537.

20. Crane GE: Pseudoparkinsonism and tardive dyskinesia. *Arch Neurol* 27:426–430, 1972.

21. Klawans HL: The pharmacology of tardive dyskinesias. *Am J Psychiatry* 130:82–86, 1973.

22. Davis KL, Berger PA, Hollister LE: Tardive dyskinesia and depressive illness. *Psychopharmacol Commun* 2:125–130, 1976.

23. Rosenbaum AH, Niven RG, Hanson NP, et al: Tardive dyskinesia: Relationship with a primary affective disorder. *Dis Nerv Syst* 38:423–427, 1977.

4 Epidemiology of Tardive Dyskinesia: Part 2

James M. Smith
John M. Kane

There is considerable interest now in prevalence of tardive dyskinesia from both a medical and clinical point of view, and questions about prevalence are central to any discussion of tardive dyskinesia. In fact, the FDA is currently considering a requirement to include incidence and/or prevalence figures for all side effects in the package inserts for psychotropics and possibly for all drugs. If they include this kind of information regarding tardive dyskinesia, it will have dramatic impact.

The high interest in risk factors related to tardive dyskinesia is based on two considerations: first, since there is no satisfactory treatment for tardive dyskinesia, it would be clinically useful to be aware of which patients are more likely to get this disorder so that some active steps in preventing these people from getting it might be taken (see also Chapter 14); second, there is the hope that if more is learned about risk factors and why some individuals or some types of individuals or patients subjected to certain types of treatments are more at risk, the pathophysiology of this disorder might be better understood.

Among the risk factors generally regarded as having a sound empirical base are: age, length of neuroleptic treatment, cumulative dose of neuroleptics, and organicity. There seems to be a recent proliferation of short review articles in which these risk factors generally are taken for granted. Among those risk factors for which data usually are equivocal are: sex, prior antiparkinson drug use, history of prior neuroleptic-induced extrapyramidal side effects (EPS), prior history of ECT, insulin shock, or lobotomy, abnormal EEG, and polypharmacy. Our review of the data on a number of these topics found that some of the risk factors once regarded as very significant may no longer have an empirical base.

PREVALENCE

It was assumed that in the more than 20 years since tardive dyskinesia was discovered that the system of obtaining prevalence estimates would be finely tuned and a fairly clear idea of how many people are actually getting tardive dyskinesia, or at least how many people have tardive dyskinesia at a point in time, would be known. In reviewing the prevalence in 56 samples reported between 1959 and 1979, this has been found to be far from true. The range of prevalence for the eight studies reported in 1979 is 3.5%[1] to 41.3%.[2] In fact, the standard deviation for the studies reported in the 1970s is 30% higher than the standard deviation of earlier studies. Despite this variability, the regression line indicates there is a clear trend toward increasing prevalence in the later studies. The average prevalence for the studies reported in the 1960s is approximately 15%, while the average prevalence for the studies reported in the 1970s is 24%, and this is a statistically significant difference.

There are several major factors affecting prevalence estimates. The first is the method of assessment. Different investigators have different ways of determining whether a patient has abnormal movements. One of the early studies used a questionnaire asking ward staff to write down the names of any patients they thought had movements typical of tardive dyskinesia. Obviously, by taking that tack the prevalence estimate is going to be rather small, because people are not going to volunteer very many patients' names. The second factor is the variety of rating scales. A third factor will be the treatment characteristics of the population studied. Clearly, patients with little exposure to neuroleptics will have a lower prevalence. And finally there are demographic characteristics, ie, age and sex. The effects of these variables on prevalence rates can be very significant. For example, if women between the ages of 70 and 90 in a state hospital are studied, a much higher prevalence will be found than if young men aged 20 to 35 in an outpatient clinic are studied. And in all the prevalence studies, some of the inconsistency results from variation in one or more of these factors.

ASSESSMENT

Gardos and Cole have reviewed some of the methods of assessment that have been used in evaluating tardive dyskinesia.[3] In addition, a variety of physiologic techniques, ie, electromyography, piezoelectric recording, and tremography, have been used to quantify the symptoms of tardive dyskinesia. These are not widely used because frequently the movements themselves do not adapt very well to that methodology. They also require a fair amount of equipment, and demand technical sophistication from the investigators as well as cooperation on the part of the patients. So, although they have been used in some studies, they are not widely used.

Many of the early studies used frequency counts, and this works very well in evaluating a symptom like flycatcher tongue; observation over a period of minutes can be made, counting how many times the patient sticks out his tongue. One problem with this method is that some movements do not lend themselves readily to frequency counts. There is also the risk that while counting the frequency of tongue protrusions, the patient could develop marked jaw movements, which would obscure the tongue protrusions and artifactually alter the rating. Frequency counts could be zero while the patient still has severe symptoms.

Finally, there are rating scales that have recently been used to measure tardive dyskinesia. Doctor Crane developed one of the first scales but this is not used very much now. In many of the recent studies, the Abnormal Involuntary Movement Scale (AIMS) (see Appendix 2), developed by the Psychopharmacology Research Branch of NIMH, has appeared as the standard rating scale for tardive dyskinesia. It has seven body area items, a global rating, and three additional ratings. This is the scale used in all of our studies. It has been found satisfactory, but has its limitations. Another scale was developed by Doctor Simpson and this is much more detailed than the AIMS, which provides global ratings of severity of movements in seven body areas. The Simpson scale is very specific in rating movements in each area. This scale rates more specific details, ie, rotation of the arm as opposed to tremor or gross athetoid movement of the fingers. It has some advantages, particularly in evaluating response to medication, but for simple prevalence surveys a scale like this can be difficult to work with.

Doctor Chouinard has developed a scale similar to the Abnormal

Involuntary Movement Scale but which differs from the AIMS in attempting to separate severity from frequency of movements. Using the AIMS, a patient with severe but infrequent movements would probably get the same rating as one who has mild but constant movements. With Chouinard's scale these two factors will be separated so that each movement is rated in a matrix, one part of the matrix being the severity of the movement and the other part of the matrix being the frequency of the movement. Then, from this matrix a precise rating is achieved. Gerlach has produced a very complex scale and there is a tardive dyskinesia scale developed by Robert Smith.

A look at those studies utilizing a severity scale (as opposed to the studies using just a nominal scale, which would rate only presence or absence of tardive dyskinesia) finds that the studies using scales that actually rate each movement show a higher prevalence than is found in studies involving only a yes/no decision. The prevalence in the studies where a scale was used was 24.4% compared to 13.9% in those studies where a scale was not employed. The difference in prevalence in studies that used scales is significant, even if only those studies conducted in the 1970s are considered. This suggests that the higher prevalence rates seen in later studies is not merely artifact due to the employment of rating scales, which were not utilized in the earlier studies.

It would be nice if all studies, which used a rating scale, arrived at similar prevalence estimates in similar samples but, unfortunately, this is not the case. Our literature review suggests that even when rating scales are used, the prevalence rates found in these studies are not consistent. One reason is that when a scale is used, the prevalence rate depends upon an arbitrary definition of where on the scale the ratings are divided into dyskinesia and nondyskinesia groups. That is, one level of abnormal movement is severe enough to be included in the dyskinesia group while another level is not. If it is decided that to include a person in the dyskinetic group, he must have a rating of a certain level on a certain symptom, then the prevalence figure is very much dependent upon what degree of severity is required for inclusion. Our own data indicate that if a criterion of a mild rating is chosen, an average rating of mild on one of those first seven items on the AIMS, prevalence is in the upper 60s.[4] On the other hand, if a stringent tack is taken and where only the most severe level of abnormal movements is going to qualify for inclusion in the dyskinetic group, then the prevalence is under 10%.

One thing to be careful about is not to diagnose a patient as having tardive dyskinesia simply because he has abnormal movements. There are many conditions that can produce abnormal movements (see Chapters 1, 5, 8, and 10). Thus, although a patient may demonstrate abnormal movements, this is not to be considered a diagnosis of tardive dyskinesia because these movements could arise from a variety of factors, and the diagnosis of tardive dyskinesia requires a careful case review, a genetic history, and evaluation of clinical signs and symptoms. It is certainly unwise to make an individual diagnosis merely on the basis of rating scale data.

RISK FACTORS

A variety of designs have been used to evaluate risk factors for tardive dyskinesia. The first one is to select a group that has the risk factor, eg, patients with lobotomies, and another group that does not have the risk factor, patients without lobotomies, and these ideally should be matched on critical variables, ie, age and sex. Once these risk groups are defined, the percentage of dyskinetic patients in each group is determined. That is one approach. If the group that had lobotomy has a higher prevalence of dyskinesia than the group without previous lobotomy, then it can be concluded that lobotomy predisposes to tardive dyskinesia.

A second design is to select a group that has tardive dyskinesia by some criterion and a second group that does not have tardive dyskinesia, and then look at the percent of each group who display the particular risk factor of interest. Thus, out of 100 patients who have tardive dyskinesia matched by age and sex with 100 patients that do not have tardive dyskinesia, the prevalence of lobotomy is 70% in the former group and 20% in the latter. Therefore, there is the suggestion that lobotomy is a risk factor.

The third approach is the multiple regression approach. This is a statistical approach to determine which variables differentiate groups or which variables highly relate one group to another. The caution with this method is that studies should be done as Chouinard does, with large samples, and not with 15 or 20 subjects. This can be a very dangerous approach when very small numbers of subjects are used, since the correlations obtained are unstable.

The underlying concern with all of these approaches to risk factors is that all are retrospective correlational studies. That is, they demonstrate what goes with what. But the problem with interpretation is the problem of the chicken and the egg. That is to say, do people with tardive dyskinesia have more EEG abnormalities than people without tardive dyskinesia, because they had more EEG abnormalities to start with and, therefore, were at risk, or because tardive dyskinesia has its own associated EEG abnormalities? In other words, do they have the risk factor before the tardive dyskinesia or do they have the risk factor because of tardive dyskinesia? Until there are prospective studies where patients are observed before they develop tardive dyskinesia, this problem always will be faced.

In our literature review, some of the specific risk factors, which have been studied in connection with tardive dyskinesia are examined. The first of these are medication related; ie, there are certain factors about medication history that might be assumed to be risk factors. First, of course, is whether the patient received neuroleptics or not. There are 19 reported samples of prevalence of abnormal involuntary movements in nonneuroleptic-treated patients and controls. In only three of these 19 samples was the prevalence greater than 10%, while most were less than 5%. There is one outlier that, unfortunately, was done in 1978. This is a study by Delwaide and Desseilles[5] who found a prevalence of 36.7% in older people not receiving neuroleptics. The report implies, however, that these patients could have been treated with neuroleptics before this group saw them. The vast majority of investigators find that the prevalence of spontaneous dyskinesias is very low. In discussions of tardive dyskinesia, people often mention senile choreas, Huntington's chorea, and all the variety of neurologic disorders that may result in involuntary movements. In fact, if all those things are taken together, even in a population of psychiatric patients, a prevalence of greater than 5% will not be found.

So, although these neurologic disorders are important to consider in differential diagnosis of an individual patient, they cannot in any way account for the high prevalence values that have been found in neuroleptic-treated groups. It appears to be clear then that neuroleptics are definitely a causative factor in the development of abnormal involuntary movements.

Other treatment variables contribute to the prevalence of tardive dyskinesia. It might be expected that duration of neuroleptic treatment and cumulative dose of neuroleptics should also be positively related to the development of tardive dyskinesia. A total of 19 studies related duration of neuroleptic treatment with tardive dyskinesia. In the 19 studies, only five found a significant relationship with duration of neuroleptic treatment. And of the five, some involved relatively brief exposure to neuroleptics. For example, Crane and Smeets[6] reported a significant relationship between length of exposure and tardive dyskinesia, but the median length of treatment for their entire sample was 11 months. And the range was three fourths of a month to 28 months, which is just over two years. So, in reality, the Crane and Smeets article suggests that if a patient receives neuroleptics for two years, he is more likely to have tardive dyskinesia than if he receives them for less than one year. That is not very surprising. It would be expected that in order to develop tardive dyskinesia, there has to be a minimum exposure period.

In addition, there is a report by Heinrich and associates[7] who also found a relationship with length of treatment, but the cutoff in that study was one year. They contrasted tardive dyskinesia in patients who were treated for less than one year with those treated for more than one year, and found a significant difference. But, looking at the bulk of studies suggests there is not a linear increase in dyskinesia with length of treatment. Instead, there most likely is a threshold beyond which a lot more dyskinesia is not seen. Put another way, if a person does not develop dyskinesia within a certain amount of time, there is a good chance he will not develop it. As a matter of fact, in looking through the literature, a remarkable percentage of patients were found who developed dyskinesia within the first three to five years of treatment. This is one thing that is beginning to be realized now; signs of tardive dyskinesia will probably be found in a sizable number of patients during the first three to five years on neuroleptics.

Regarding the cumulative dose of neuroleptics, it might be expected that the more drug received over the entire course of treatment, the more likely would be the development of tardive dyskinesia. Here, also, the results are relatively disappointing. Only seven of 19 studies found a significant relationship, and in one of these the relationship was a negative one. Again, in some of the studies the cutoffs are very low. For example, in the Crane and Smeets study,[6] they cut off at 50 mg/day/year. It was not defined this way but when their data are researched, one group is found who received less than 50 mg/day/year *vs* a group who received more, and certainly a difference between these two groups then would be expected.

There has been some thought that the dose of neuroleptics may be a significant factor; that if a patient is given very high doses, he may be more susceptible to tardive dyskinesia. Two studies find a relationship between maximum dose and tardive dyskinesia,[8,9] and one study finds no relationship.[10]

Another possible risk factor studied is polypharmacy. People like to think that because polypharmacy is disapproved of, it is a risk factor for tardive dyskinesia. There are three studies[11-13] in which the patients' exposure to polypharmacy was related to tardive dyskinesia and none found a significant relationship.

Why do the studies of drug treatment variables yield such poor results? There may be many reasons. For one thing, in the duration and cumulative dose studies, in most instances it is unknown when the patients developed dyskinesia. It is possible they could have developed it very early on in treatment; and yet now they are considered as having received 5000 g of chlorpromazine, while they may have developed tardive dyskinesia after only 1000 g of chlorpromazine. And without that information, it makes the data very uncertain. Secondly, there is the problem of compliance, even with inpatients. If, over a period of ten years, a patient had been prescribed 5000 g of chlorpromazine, perhaps he actually only took 2000 g of chlorpromazine. That adds additional uncertainty to the situation. And finally, there are individual differences in absorption and excretion. These measurements are in terms of ingested amounts of drug, and blood levels of neuroleptics do not correlate well with oral dosage. It is not surprising, therefore, that the drug history data also would not correlate with tardive dyskinesia.

If neuroleptic drug history variables relate relatively poorly to prevalence or severity of tardive dyskinesia, then perhaps the patient's sensitivity to EPS is a better index of the likelihood of late developing tardive dyskinesia. One study examined this relationship directly,[14] and found no significant relationship (see also Chapter 3). Of the 18 studies relating prior use of antiparkinsonian drugs to the subsequent development of tardive dyskinesia, only five found a significant relationship.

In terms of treatment variables or risk factors that are not related to medication, the data are similarly weak. There is little indication of any significant relationship of tardive dyskinesia to prior lobotomy, ECT, or insulin coma treatment. Our review of the literature indicated that only 3 of 20 comparisons involving these treatments were statistically significant. History of neurologic disease or clinical evidence of neurologic dysfunction (abnormal EEG or CT scan) also showed little relationship, with only 5 of 20 studies having significant findings.

The findings are more convincing, however, regarding certain demographic factors in relationship to tardive dyskinesia. The review found 13 of 30 studies showing a statistically significant relationship between age and tardive dyskinesia. Furthermore, 10 of the 17 studies that did not find a significant relationship involved samples from a restricted age range. Increasing age is related to greater susceptibility for developing tardive dyskinesia.

The available data also show a relationship between females and a greater prevalence of tardive dyskinesia. In nearly 90% of the samples, which presented data on male and female prevalence, females had the greater prevalence, although the male/female difference was not statistically significant in all of these studies. In contrast to the often cited 2:1 female:male ratio, the combined ratio in all of these samples, involving more than 15,000 patients, was only slightly greater than 1.5:1. The data also strongly suggest females are more prone to develop more severe forms of the disorder. Whether these sex differences are the result of true biological differences or merely different treatment histories remains to be determined.

There are three recently mentioned, and as yet unconfirmed, risk factors that may prove worthwhile investigating. The first is the number of prior neuroleptic-free intervals in the patient's medication history. Ironically, the greater the number of such intervals, the more likely the patient will be to develop irreversible tardive dyskinesia. The second is prior history of depressive symptoms, which has been positively related to tardive dyskinesia (see also Chapter 3). The third is overall treatment refractoriness. There appears to be a positive relationship between lack of clinical improvement (as indicated by scores on rating scales or rate of discharge) and prevalence or severity of tardive dyskinesia. It should be emphasized that, at the present time, these are mere conjectures based on very limited, uncontrolled studies, and it remains to be seen whether these factors will be found to be significant in larger, controlled studies.

The aim of our review of the literature, in relationship to risk factors, was to separate fact from fantasy. We owe it to ourselves, and to our patients, to be perfectly clear about what has been demonstrated empirically and what has not. Unfortunately, when these data are reviewed systematically, the latter far outweigh the former.

REFERENCES

1. Alexopoulos GS: Lack of complaints in schizophrenics with tardive dyskinesia. *J Nerv Ment Dis* 167:125–127, 1979.

2. Smith JM, Kucharski LT, Eblen C, et al: An assessment of tardive dyskinesia in schizophrenic outpatients. *Psychopharmacology* 64:99–104, 1979.

3. Gardos G, Cole JO, LaBrie RA: The assessment of tardive dyskinesia. *Arch Gen Psychiatry* 34:1206–1212, 1977.

4. Smith JM, Oswald WT, Kucharski LT, et al: Tardive dyskinesia: age and sex differences in hospitalized schizophrenics. *Psychopharmacology* 58:207–211, 1978.

5. Delwaide PJ, Desseilles M: Spontaneous buccolinguofacial dyskinesia in the elderly. *Acta Neurol Scand* 56:256–262, 1977.

6. Crane, GE, Smeets RA: Tardive dyskinesia and drug therapy in geriatric patients. *Arch Gen Psychiatry* 30:341–343, 1974.

7. Heinrich K, Wegener I, Bender HJ: Spate extrapyramidale hyperkinesen bei neuroleptischer langzeit-therapie. *Pharmakopsychiatr Neuropsychopharmakol* 1:169–195, 1968.

8. Smith RC, Strizich M, Klass D: Drug history and tardive dyskinesia. *Am J Psychiatry* 135:1402–1403, 1978.

9. Crane GE: Factors predisposing to drug-induced neurologic effects, in Forrest IS, Carr CJ, Usdin E (eds): *Phenothiazines and Structurally Related Drugs*. New York, Raven Press, 1974, pp 269–279.

10. Gardos G, Cole JO, LaBrie RA: Drug variables in etiology of tardive dyskinesia: application of discriminant function analysis. *Neuropsychopharmacology* 1:147–155, 1977.

11. Jus A, Pineau R, LaChance R, et al: Epidemiology of tardive dyskinesia: Part II. *Dis Nerv Syst* 37:257–261, 1976.

12. Demars JPCA: Neuromuscular effects of long-term phenothiazine medication, electroconvulsive therapy and leucotomy. *J Nerv Ment Dis* 143:73–79, 1966.

13. Simpson GM, Varga E, Lee JH, et al: Tardive dyskinesia and psychotropic drug history. *Psychopharmacology* 58:117–124, 1978.

14. Jus A, Pineau R, LaChance R, et al: Epidemiology of tardive dyskinesia: Part I. *Dis Nerv Syst* 37:210–214, 1976.

5 Practical Diagnosis of Common Involuntary Movement Disorders

Luciano M. Modesti

Movements are defined as involuntary when they cannot be prevented, attenuated, or suppressed at will. As such, they disturb rest and interfere considerably with the initiation, duration, completion, and precision of attempted volitional acts. Since medieval times, when involuntary motor manifestations were attributed to demonic influence, parental sins, or insanity, some understanding has been gained regarding the pathogenesis of abnormal movements but much remains to be learned. At present, it is universally accepted that involuntary movements or dyskinesias are clinical expressions of functional disorders of the basal ganglia and their various connections, but anatomical and physiological investigations have elucidated but a few clinical-pathological correlations. Damage of a particular cerebral structure can seldom be linked clinically with the appearance of specific types of involuntary movements.

Attempts to reproduce dyskinesias of humans in animal models have yielded inconsistent results, probably because of the higher degree of organization of the basal ganglia in man, who has adopted an erect posture and is capable of performing a wider range of skilled movements. Lesions at different sites often cause identical movements; on the other hand, different pathological processes affecting the same structures may result in various dyskinetic syndromes. Furthermore, similar disorders may respond to different surgical lesions and, paradoxically, identical lesions will benefit different types of dyskinesia. The proliferation of etiopathogenetic theories trying to explain the clinical manifestations of basal ganglia disease is in inverse proportion to our actual physiological understanding; that is to say, our present knowledge of the pathology encountered in patients with movement disorders cannot be integrated into well-defined anatomical, physiological, and clinical entities.

Recent advances in experimental and clinical neuropharmacology have crystallized the role of the neurotransmitters in all intercellular connections responsible for the multiple and complex functions of the nervous system. The action of the neurotransmitters seems to be directed toward the preservation of an appropriate balance between excitation and inhibition among the neurons involved in motor control. The exact pharmacological mechanism underlying abnormal movements, whether in the form of excess or depletion of specific neurotransmitters or of hypersensitivity of certain cells to a normal amount of chemical transmitters, is still elusive. Movement disorders may well represent overactivity of certain areas of the motor system in the absence of the controlling influence of other diseased structures with the functional manifestation of release, excessive facilitation, or disorganized integration of sensory signals. The time-honored correlations of Parkinson's disease with lesions of the nigrostriatal system, Huntington's chorea with degeneration of the caudate, and hemiballismus with a localized lesion of the subthalamic nucleus, are oversimplifications that are no longer acceptable. At the present stage of our knowledge, we can only state that abnormal movement disorders are the clinical expression of nonspecific changes affecting the anatomical, physiological, and chemical properties of the basal ganglia and their connecting pathways.

The foregoing discussion leads to the obvious conclusions that involuntary movements can be appreciated only on the basis of individual symptoms and signs and that an etiological classification, although desirable, is not feasible. Conventionally, all dyskinesias are classified in descriptive terms, according to their distinctive morphological features. In many involuntary movement disorders, to see is to diagnose. The patient's detailed personal and family history must be obtained, with particular emphasis regarding instances and types of motor disorders and neurological diseases in distant and near relatives, birth trauma, use of drugs or alcohol, previous central nervous system infections, head injury, seizures, and occupational or accidental exposure to toxic agents. Keen and prolonged observation of the patient and his relatives should be followed by a detailed description of the movements. Their location, amplitude, rhythm, speed, and duration should be carefully recorded, together with any speech disturbance. Particular attention should be devoted to the influence upon the movements of stress, posture, rest, distraction, ambulation, and voluntary motion. As a general rule, all involuntary movements cease during sleep and become more pronounced during observation and testing. At this point, a complete neurological examination is carried out for detection of associated organic deficits like dementia, papilledema, nystagmus, spasticity, rigidity, paresis, pathologic reflexes, and dysphasia.

Involuntary movements will be described here according to their morphological and dynamic patterns without reference to the underlying pathological process. Not uncommonly, different types of dyskinesias may in time merge into one another or be present simultaneously in the same patient. Disorders of movements of clear organic origin, ie, myoclonus and seizures, are omitted in this presentation, as are habit spasm and tics, which usually are manifestations of obsessive compulsive neurosis.

INVOLUNTARY MOVEMENTS

Tremors

Tremors are the involuntary movements most often encountered. These consist of rhythmic, alternating contractions of opposing muscles with variable amplitude and rate of oscillation. A barely noticeable, low-amplitude physiological tremor can become accentuated under emotional stress, fatigue, cold weather, and excessive use of coffee, alcohol or tobacco. Senile tremor of the elderly is an exaggeration of the physiological tremor and affects mostly the head, neck, lips, tongue, and arms. There are no other neurological abnormalities.

Pathological tremors are classified according to their relationship to voluntary activity. Resting tremor is pathognomonic of Parkinson's disease and in this circumstance is usually accompanied by bradykinesis, rigidity, facial amimicry, short-stepped gait, and stooped posture. In some parkinsonian patients, the tremor is the most distressing symptom and, unfortunately, the least sensitive to levodopa therapy. Parkinsonian tremor begins on one side and may remain unilateral, but generally it spreads to the opposite side after a variable period of time. The most commonly affected parts are the tongue, hands, and feet. Resting tremor disappears only temporarily during action.

Heredofamilial or essential tremor is instead a postural type. It is often mistaken for a symptom of parkinsonism, from which it should be carefully differentiated since it carries a much less serious long-term prognosis. Essential tremor is brought about by sustained posture, like holding the outstretched arms forward. It is usually absent or minimally present at rest. Familial tremor may be noticed already in the early adult years, may progress with age, and become functionally and socially embarrassing. At this stage, writing, feeding, and other skilled movements are seriously impaired. Characteristically, this type of tremor is alleviated by alcohol and beta-adrenergic blocking agents like propranolol. Very similar to essential tremor is the tremor associated with lithium therapy for manic depressive illness. Most patients will develop postural tremor if given high doses of this medication.

Pathological processes of a different nature, ie, trauma, infections, multiple sclerosis, tumors, and phenytoin toxicity, may manifest with intention or cerebellar tremor, which predominantly affects the proximal muscles. The amplitude is wide and much more accentuated toward the termination of the movement near the target. This type of tremor is best demonstrated by asking the patient to perform the finger-to-nose test. Intention tremor is related to lesions of the superior cerebellar peduncle. In severe cases of multiple sclerosis, the disorganized arm movements are very disabling and can be alleviated only by stereotaxic thalamotomy.

Chorea

The quick, darting, rapid, and unpredictable jerks of chorea give the impression of a fidgety, purposeless activity. Any part of the body, including the face, tongue, pharynx, and larynx, can be involved at irregular intervals. Choreic movements are brief, pleomorphic, and seldom completed. They are aptly described as a caricature of normal movements. Emotional lability and impulsive behavior may complicate the motor hyperkinesis. The postrheumatic form of Sydenham's chorea of childhood and adolescence is self-limiting, and usually subsides in a few months without serious sequelae. Similarly benign are the chorea gravidarum and those choreiform syndromes complicating treatment with oral contraceptives, phenytoin, amphetamines, and anticholinergic drugs. Much more serious implications are carried in the hereditary disorder, Huntington's chorea. In this syndrome, the movements are slower and more bizarre, especially in the face and upper limbs. Progressive intellectual deterioration may precede or follow the choreic manifestations and eventually leads to total dementia. In the absence of a firm family history, the diagnosis can only be presumptive.

Hemiballismus

Hemiballismus is the expression of a vascular or neoplastic lesion affecting the subthalamic nucleus and its connections with the globus pallidus. The abnormal motor hyperactivity is similar to that of chorea, but much more violent. The proximal muscles of the affected limbs are animated by incessant, exhausting, flinging and throwing motions. The typical flail-like pattern makes the diagnosis quite obvious. Hemichorea and hemiballismus are considered by many as different degrees of the same syndrome rather than as two separate entities. Therapy with haloperidol or fluphenazine usually is beneficial, but sometimes thalamotomy is indicated in those cases that do not respond to medical management.

Athetosis

The hallmark of athetosis (mobile spasm) is the presence of slow, writhing, relatively continuous postural changes in the distal limbs. Hands and fingers are affected most frequently by repetitive episodes of extreme twisting, which a normal person cannot reproduce. The forearm is held pronated with flexion of the wrist and hyperextension of the fingers. Since this dyskinesia is often related to birth injury, there also may be spasticity, paresis, and mental retardation. Other etiological factors are: cerebral trauma, anoxic encephalopathy, and carbon monoxide intoxication. Status marmoratus of the putamen is the pathological substrate of the perinatal form related to anoxia (cerebral palsy with double athetosis). The movements of athetosis are highly variable; consequently, the difference from chorea and dystonia at times may become indistinct. This may be one reason why many authors prefer to adopt the term choreoathetosis in those cases where the movement patterns cannot be clearly differentiated.

Dystonia

Dystonia is a disorder of posture induced by slow, sustained alternating contractions and relaxation of agonist and antagonist muscles. As a result, the body assumes grotesque contortions and when the contractions of a muscle group are predominant and prolonged, irreducible fixed contractures occur. Symptomatic torsion dystonia may be one clinical aspect of many neurological diseases with a known pathological basis, ie, Wilson's disease, cerebrovascular insult, anoxia at birth, head trauma, and Huntington's chorea.

In the idiopathic form of dystonia musculorum deformans the cause is unknown. There is no intellectual or neurological deficit, and no specific pathological or laboratory abnormalities have been identified. The childhood onset type is generally inherited and manifests as early disturbance of gait with progression toward generalized dystonia in a few years and ultimately severe disability. By contrast, the adult torsion dystonia is characterized by onset in the arms and axial structures and usually by absence of progression. In some subjects, the dystonic movements may remain localized in one limb or other body part. These forms are called segmental or focal dystonias. Examples are the so-called occupational cramps, blepharospasm, oromandibular dystonias, pharyngolaryngeal distonias, and the better known spasmodic torticollis. A common feature to all these syndromes is the presence of dystonic posture due to recurrent and sustained spasm of the involved muscles, very similar to that observed in the idiopathic dystonia musculorum deformans.

The question whether these conditions are of organic or psychogenic nature, or both, has been debated for a long time. Several objective findings support the view that focal dystonias are of organic origin. They may occur in members of families in which focal dystonias or dystonia musculorum deformans developed in other subjects. Focal dystonias may appear following use of psychotropic drugs. Often they respond dramatically to stereotaxic surgery. Lastly, they may be part of the clinical picture of dystonia musculorum deformans or be the initial feature of that illness.

Tardive Dyskinesia

A discussion on involuntary movements would be incomplete without some comments on tardive dyskinesias. This topic is extensively reviewed in this publication, but a few considerations here will emphasize some paradoxical phenomena we are confronting in the diagnosis and treatment of these peculiar syndromes.

Tardive dyskinesias, the various forms of dystonia, and the involuntary movements complicating levodopa therapy for parkinsonism, all share not only clinical similarities but also a broad pharmacological common denominator. The differential diagnosis of these syndromes may be difficult, but essentially it is based upon a careful history of previous drug intake and by eliminating any drug to see if the symptoms disappear. It may be helpful to recall that drug-induced involuntary movements seem to occur more frequently in elderly female patients, after prolonged treatment. Tardive dyskinesias are encountered during protracted therapy with phenothiazines and butyrophenones. Interestingly enough, these very same drugs are used with success for control of abnormal motor manifestations caused by the same or related agents, and for relief of spontaneously occurring abnormal movements like torticollis, hemiballismus, and chorea.

There are other puzzling aspects of the dyskinesias which thus far appear to lack plausible explanation. A rare complication of stereotaxic thalamotomy for relief of parkinsonian tremor is the insurgence of various dyskinetic syndromes, which may respond to phenothiazines and haloperidol. Previously operated upon parkinsonian patients do not develop levodopa-induced dyskinesia on the side of the previous tremor that benefited from surgery. All of these disconcerting observations implicate an uncertain role of dopamine and other cerebral amines in the genesis of abnormal movements. It only can be speculated now whether movement disorders are due to increased synthesis of dopamine, to blocking effect upon cerebral dopamine receptors, to altered sensitivity of denervated striatal neurons, or to the possible existence of a heterogeneous population of cells with different pharmacological properties.

The obvious indiscriminate influence of cerebral amines over a variety of abnormal movements indicates a very delicate and complex biochemical mechanism, which is still poorly understood. The basal ganglia are slowly giving away some of their physiological secrets. Once the intricate mosaic is completed, the distressing and frustrating problem of involuntary movements will become another glorious chapter in the history of the highest medical achievement.

SUGGESTED READING

Brain Lord: Extrapyramidal syndromes, in Walton, JN (ed): *Diseases of the Nervous System,* ed 8. New York, Oxford University Press, 1977, pp 569–614.

Duvoisin R: Clinical diagnosis of the dyskinesias. *Med Clin North Am* 56:1321–1341, 1972.

Marsden CD: The neuropharmacology of abnormal involuntary movement disorders (the dyskinesias), in Williams D (ed): *Modern Trends in Neurology,* vol 6. Woburn, MA, Butterworths, 1975, pp 141–146.

Yahr MD: Involuntary movements, in Critchley M et al (eds): *Scientific Foundations of Neurology.* Philadelphia, F.A. Davis Co, 1972, pp 83–88.

6 The Rational Use of Antipsychotic Drugs

Donald M. Pirodsky

Since there really is no overall effective treatment for tardive dyskinesia at this time, the best way to decrease the incidence of this syndrome is via primary prevention. In other words, preventing it from occurring in the first place. And, short of that, we at least hope for early detection, because the earlier the syndrome is detected and the antipsychotic drugs are discontinued, the greater the chance of remission. Some general guidelines concerning the use of antipsychotic drugs are essential, therefore, in order to achieve or maintain the optimal benefits of these drugs, as well as decrease the risk of their side effects. Keep in mind that these are guidelines and not hard and fast rules. They are intended to advise the clinician in the use of medications and to avoid some of the common pitfalls often seen in the prescription of these drugs.

First, it is important to know when, or when not, to use antipsychotics. These are potent drugs and their use should be reserved for major psychiatric disorders. Table 6-1 lists their indications. It is a relatively extensive list and the really primary indications are the first two, schizophrenia and mania (principally schizophrenia, both acute and chronic). In terms of improvement, roughly 75% of newly diagnosed schizophrenics can be expected to respond to antipsychotics. Improvement in the thought disorder is seen, and also the degree of agitation or withdrawal. Since schizophrenia is the main indication, the guidelines referred to here are essentially for use in its treatment.

Table 6-1
Antipsychotic Drug Indications

1. Schizophrenia
2. Mania
3. Acute organic brain syndrome (delirium)
4. Chronic organic brain syndrome (dementia)
5. Psychoses and behavioral problems associated with mental retardation
6. Depression
7. Other indications
   a. Gilles de la Tourette's syndrome
   b. Nausea and vomiting
   c. Intractable hiccups
   d. Huntington's chorea

Lithium is the treatment of choice for mania. But lithium has a relatively slow onset of action, taking about seven days to exert its full effect. And while waiting for lithium to exert its effect, antipsychotics are often a useful adjunct. After the mania is under control, the antipsychotic agent then can be tapered and discontinued, and the patient maintained on lithium. Lithium is effective in about 80% of manic patients. For the 20% who do not respond to lithium, the treatment of choice is an antipsychotic agent alone.

An acute organic brain syndrome or delirium may be seen following surgery. For example, postcardiotomy delirium occurs when patients are on the heart/lung pump for prolonged periods of time. This may also be seen secondary to metabolic problems, ie, increased BUN, increased serum ammonia level, or hyponatremia. Frequently, these people will be quietly confused and will require no treatment other than environmental manipulation and correction of the underlying cause. But at times, delirium can be truly life threatening. For example, postoperatively, patients may try to extubate themselves, pull out their IVs, or walk out of the Intensive Care Unit. When medication is needed to control delirium until the underlying cause is corrected, an antipsychotic drug is indicated. The sedative drugs, the barbiturates and the benzodiazepines, will often aggravate a delirium. An exception to this would be the delirium secondary to alcohol withdrawal. For delirium tremens the benzodiazepines are the drugs of choice.

In institutions, people with dementia often become irritable with minimal provocation and may become assaultive or belligerent to nursing staff and other patients on the unit. When environmental manipulation does not prove useful, the treatment of choice if medication is needed is an antipsychotic agent, generally in low doses.

With psychoses and behavioral problems associated with mental retardation, medication should be thought of only as an adjunct to any overall treatment plan. It is not indicated for all patients with mental retardation, but only for those who manifest severe self-abusive behavior, unprovoked assaultive/aggressive behavior, autistic-like behaviors (stereotyped, repetitive, self-stimulatory behaviors), or uncontrollable hyperactivity. When a medication is needed to control these symptoms, the antipsychotics are the drugs of choice.

Depression is also included on the list, but is not really an indication. In other words, antipsychotics are not the drugs of choice in treating depression per se. They can make some depressions worse, particularly the sedating antipsychotics like chlorpromazine and thioridazine. However, the combination of an antipsychotic and a tricyclic antidepressant is often useful for psychotic depressions, and can be more effective than the tricyclic alone. We frequently find that the antipsychotic helps the delusions, hallucinations, and agitation that often go along with psychotic depressions.

Another indication listed in Table 6-1 is for Gilles de la Tourette's syndrome, which has been found to respond to antipsychotic drugs, specifically haloperidol (see Chapter 10). Prochlorperazine (Compazine) is the most commonly used drug for nausea and vomiting. However, many people are not aware it is a phenothiazine. Other antipsychotic drugs also have strong antiemetic effects. For example, chlorpromazine and haloperidol are potent in this respect. An important aspect of this indication is that some patients with chronic gastrointestinal problems are maintained on low doses of prochlorperazine, or a combination drug that contains prochlorperazine (eg, Combid). If these drugs are continued for long periods of time, one risks the development of tardive dyskinesia (see also Chapters 11 and 14).

For intractable hiccups, chlorpromazine has been reported to be effective when more conservative measures fail.

Last on the list is Huntington's chorea. Unfortunately there is nothing that will reverse the basic neuropathological process of Huntington's chorea, but antipsychotics by virtue of their dopamine receptor blockade can help in controlling the involuntary movements of this disorder.

The guidelines for clinical use of these drugs are outlined in Table 6-2. First, make an accurate diagnosis. Ascertain that the symptoms the patient has are going to be relieved by the medication. Again, these are potent drugs and should not be used unless there is a clear-cut indication.

Table 6-2
Summary of Guidelines for Clinical Use

---

1. Make an accurate diagnosis.
2. Choice of drug. Consider the following:
   a. Patient's prior drug response history.
   b. Family drug response history.
   c. Side effects.
3. Do not confuse potency with efficacy.
4. Become thoroughly familiar with several drugs.
5. Initiate treatment with a single drug.
   a. Small test dose.
   b. Starting dose.
   c. Gradually increase into effective antipsychotic range.
6. Dosage Schedule.
   a. Divided doses initially.
   b. Shift to once or twice daily schedule.
7. After improvement, gradually taper dose to maintenance level.
8. Decide how long to continue medication.
9. If refractory to one drug, switch to a more potent drug of the same class or to a drug in another class.
10. Avoid polypharmacy.
11. Use antiparkinsonian agents judiciously.

When a diagnosis is made (assume a diagnosis of schizophrenia), then a decision of which drug to use must follow. Table 6-3 lists the various antipsychotic drugs along with their usual dose ranges. There are five different classes of antipsychotics: the phenothiazines, of which there are three subgroups, the aliphatics, piperidines, and piperazines; the thioxanthenes; the butyrophenones; the dihydroindolones; and the dibenzoxazepines. With five different classes, choosing a drug can become relatively complicated. How can the prescribing physician narrow down this choice and come up with a more suitable drug for any given patient?

Whenever possible, the choice of an antipsychotic agent should be based on the patient's prior drug response history. For example, if a schizophrenic patient has responded to acetophenazine (Tindal) in the past, that is the drug that should be tried first. Likewise, if he or she has

Table 6-3
Equivalent Doses and Usual Daily Dose Ranges
of Oral Forms of Antipsychotic Agents*

Generic Name	Trade Name	Approximate Equivalent Dose (mg)	Usual Daily Dose Range (mg/day)	
			Acute	*Maintenance*
Phenothiazines				
Aliphatic				
chlorpromazine	Thorazine	100	300–1600	100 – 400
triflupromazine	Vesprin	25	75–150	25–100
Piperidine				
mesoridazine	Serentil	50	150–400	50–200
piperacetazine	Quide	10	40–160	20–50
thioridazine	Mellaril	100	300–800	100–400
Piperazine				
acetophenazine	Tindal	20	60–120	40–80
butaperazine	Repoise	10	30–100	10–40
carphenazine	Proketazine	25	75–400	25–150
fluphenazine	Prolixin Permitil	2	6–60	2–8
perphenazine	Trilafon	8	16–64	8–24
prochlorperazine	Compazine	15	50–150	20–60
trifluoperazine	Stelazine	5	15–60	5–15
Thioxanthenes				
chlorprothixene	Taractan	100	300–600	75–400
thiothixene	Navane	5	15–60	6–30
Butyrophenones				
haloperidol	Haldol	2	6–100	2–8
Dihydroindolones				
molindone	Moban Lidone	10	40–225	15–60
Dibenzoxazepines				
loxapine	Loxitane Daxolin	15	50–250	20–75

*By permission from Pirodsky DM: *Primer of Clinical Psychopharmacology: A Practical Guide.* Garden City, NY, Medical Examination Publishing Co Inc, 1981.

responded to thiothixene (Navane), then that should be the drug of first choice.

More often than not, however, there is no personal drug response history. It may be the patient's first episode. When such is the case, the choice of drug can be based on the drug response history of the patient's family, specifically a blood relative. And there is a reason for this. All of these drugs in equivalent doses are effective agents for any given individual. However, patients respond to drugs differently. For example, some respond better to haloperidol than to chlorpromazine, and vice versa, which may be related to such factors as absorption of the drug, metabolism of the drug, or perhaps even differences in receptor blockade. These differences can be genetically determined. So, whenever possible, base the choice of the drug on the family drug response history when a personal one is not available.

In many instances, neither one of these guidelines is available. A choice can be made based on the side effects that these drugs produce. Of all the possible side effects, the main concerns should be extrapyramidal symptoms, excessive sedation, anticholinergic effects, and postural hypotension.

The aliphatic and piperidine phenothiazines can be thought of as being high in sedation, high in anticholinergic activity, and having a greater tendency to produce postural hypotension than all of the others listed in Table 6-3. With the piperazine phenothiazines and other classes of antipsychotics, the most common side effect is some type of extrapyramidal symptom.

There are some exceptions, eg, loxapine tends to produce a moderate degree of sedation. In general, however, these latter drugs produce extrapyramidal symptoms and have less tendency to produce excessive sedation, anticholinergic effects, and postural hypotension. Thus, for a highly agitated schizophrenic patient, substantial sedation may not be undesirable and a drug like chlorpromazine or thioridazine might be chosen. But for a withdrawn schizophrenic any more sedation than necessary would not allow him or her to participate in the general treatment milieu of the ward. Thus, in this case the drug of choice might be fluphenazine, thiothixene, or haloperidol, which have less sedation.

For elderly patients or patients who have cardiovascular problems, drugs that cause postural hypotension should be used only with due caution and careful clinical monitoring. The drug chosen is the one that is felt will give the patient the least side effects, since it is known they are all effective antipsychotic agents.

Although these drugs vary in potency (see Table 6-3), they are all effective agents when given in equivalent doses. Potency should not be confused with efficacy. How can the choice be narrowed down further? It is unlikely for clinicians to be totally familiar with all of these drugs. Therefore, it is recommended that the physician choose one or two drugs from each of the subgroups of the phenothiazines and one drug from each of the other classes and become thoroughly familiar with those agents.

To summarize, after a diagnosis is made, a drug is chosen based on the patient's prior drug response history or on the family drug response history, when the former is not available. When neither one is available, the drug of choice is the one with the fewest troublesome side effects. Do not confuse potency with efficacy, and become thoroughly familiar with several drugs.

For our discussion, a diagnosis of schizophrenia has been made and a drug has been chosen. The next step is to initiate treatment. Treatment is always started with a single drug. Although it is not absolutely necessary, a small test dose of the drug should be given first, ie, 25 to 50 mg of chlorpromazine or the equivalent dose of another drug. This is a nice way to check for any adverse effects, but may not always be practical, ie, with an acutely agitated patient. If no adverse effects are observed two hours after a test dose is given, then the dose can be increased into the effective antipsychotic range.

The rate at which the dose is increased depends on the clinical condition of the patient. As a rough guideline, however, 300 to 400 mg of chlorpromazine a day (or the equivalent dose of another drug) could be given initially and the dose gradually increased every two to three days until an adequate therapeutic response is effected or troublesome side effects intervene. This generally is done within a six-week period or less, but patients with exacerbations of chronic schizophrenia may need up to a three-month treatment period before the response should be judged. A young, acutely agitated schizophrenic could be started with a higher dose and the dose increased more rapidly. On the other hand, an older patient, or perhaps one who is less agitated, could be started with a lower dose and the dose increased more slowly.

The dose ranges listed in Table 6-3 are approximate or usual ranges. They are not absolute upper limits. The important thing to keep in mind is that the individual needs of the patient have to be taken into account. This is particularly true at the higher end of the spectrum. More is known about the minimum effective dose levels of antipsychotic drugs than is known about the upper dose levels. In terms of the minimum dose level, doses of less than 300 to 400 mg/day of chlorpromazine have not been found to be effective in the treatment of acute schizophrenia. An insufficient dose may be one reason for a patient's failure to respond; and this is one of the more common pitfalls in the use of antipsychotics. All too often, people who do not respond or who respond a little (but not optimally), are just left on that dose. They are considered either refractory or to have responded "as much as they are going to." If these drugs are to be used, patients deserve to be given a full therapeutic trial with them.

Concerning the dosage schedule for these drugs, initially a divided dose minimizes the impact of side effects and also allows for better titration. Once the therapeutic dose is established, the frequency then can be reduced. All antipsychotics are long acting, with a half-life of approximately 24 hours. Thus, they need be given no more than once or twice a day. Often, a single bedtime dose of medication is the most feasible regimen. This does two things. Giving the dose all at bedtime increases compliance and reduces the incidence of side effects. A study was done regarding compliance and showed that when an antipsychotic was prescribed qid, the compliance rate was roughly 25%. On the other hand, when it was given once a day hs, the compliance rate went up to 90%, a significant increase.

In terms of side effects, most of these drugs have some sedative activity. Thus, when a bedtime dose is prescribed, it cuts out the need to give any other medication to induce sleep and avoids unwanted daytime sedation. Also, when the dose is taken at bedtime, the blood level peaks about two hours later, which is when some extrapyramidal side effects are most likely to occur. However, extrapyramidal side effects disappear with sleep. Thus, if the blood level peaks while the patient is asleep, he is not going to experience any extrapyramidal side effects.

There is an exception, however, to this general rule of giving a single bedtime dose, and that is with elderly patients. Elderly patients may not be able to tolerate a single large bolus of one of these drugs. They may require a tid or qid schedule. In other cases, when a single hs dose is not feasible, one third of the dose can be taken in the morning and two thirds at hs, giving the majority hs to decrease daytime side effects.

As mentioned previously a 75% improvement rate can be expected in newly diagnosed schizophrenic patients. The first signs of improvement generally seen are changes in the behavior pattern and changes in the sleep pattern. They are often a good clue as to how well the patient is going to respond further along. Thus, an improved sleep pattern and a decrease in agitation, belligerence, and assaultiveness are early signs of response. Later in the course of treatment improvement in the thought disorder, delusions, and hallucinations may be seen. Although specific antipsychotic effects may be seen in as little as two days, or even earlier with rapid tranquilization techniques, optimal benefit may take up to six weeks or longer. Waiting a full six weeks will insure an adequate therapeutic trial.

Once improvement has occurred and the patient's condition has stabilized, usually between four and 12 weeks, then the dose should be decreased gradually. This is important as often a patient is left on a given dose indefinitely, which is not good practice. It increases the risk of long-term side effects, particularly tardive dyskinesia. Again, after optimal improvement is seen and the patient's condition is stabilized, consider tapering the dose over a period of weeks. Too rapid a reduction might result in a relapse; gradual tapering allows for an eventual maintenance dose. It may be that this maintenance dose is roughly one third to one fifth of the peak dose used, but again, there is considerable variation from patient to patient. So one has to rely on clinical judgment. The eventual maintenance dose should be the lowest dose that retains therapeutic gains and allows the patient to function best.

To summarize, treatment is initiated with a small test dose, a starting dose is chosen, and increased gradually into the effective antipsychotic range until optimal improvement is obtained or troublesome side effects intervene. Use divided doses initially, but for most people this should later be changed to a once or twice daily schedule. After improvement occurs, gradually taper the dose to a maintenance level.

How long should the maintenance dose be continued after remission has occurred? There are different opinions on this, but some generalizations can be made. For example, for a patient with an initial schizophrenic episode, maintenance medication can be discontinued after six to eight months, assuming that the patient's remission is stable. However, some clinicians recommend discontinuing the medication prior to six months to decrease the risk of developing tardive dyskinesia. For a patient with a second schizophrenic episode, maintenance therapy might be continued for approximately two years. If a patient has three or more episodes, maintenance therapy may be needed indefinitely. The physician has to weigh the benefit of maintenance treatment against the risk of developing tardive dyskinesia. Earlier discontinuation may be advisable. Again, there is no substitute for good clinical judgment here. Ideally, this issue of maintenance treatment should be discussed with the patient and his or her informed consent obtained (see Chapter 15).

Chronic schizophrenics should be maintained on the lowest possible dose of antipsychotic medication that will keep their symptoms in remission, and periodic attempts (at least once a year) should be made to discontinue the drugs altogether. This decreases the patients' total exposure to the drugs and allows for the early detection of any signs of tardive dyskinesia. This point cannot be stressed enough. There are also many chronic schizophrenics maintained on low doses of medication who are getting little benefit from the drug, and for these patients the drug may be safely discontinued. Again, weigh the benefits vs the risk of developing long-term side effects, and if the benefits are not substantial then the drug should be discontinued.

What can be done if a newly diagnosed schizophrenic patient does not respond well to maximally tolerated doses of an antipsychotic within six weeks (or for a chronic schizophrenic who has an acute exacerbation, within three months)? This is another common pitfall in the use of antipsychotics. All too often patients are left on medications that they are really refractory to. Sometimes clinicians are hesitant to say that a patient is refractory because there may be some improvement in his or her condition, even though it is far from optimal. Ward staff may be apprehensive about a medication change in a patient who has shown some degree of improvement (particularly an assaultive or belligerent patient). This apprehension is often transmitted to the physician. The point is not to be afraid to admit that the patient is refractory to one of these drugs (with antidepressant drugs this is done more readily). However, with schizophrenics there is a tendency to accept less than optimal gain. But, before considering a patient refractory, make sure that his lack of response is not due to either a failure to ingest or absorb the drug. Older people, in particular, may have problems with absorption. This can be detected by giving a short course of IM administration.

When, however, a patient is refractory to any given drug, switch to a more potent drug of the same class or to a drug in another class. There are a couple of reasons for this. As mentioned earlier, genetic factors may play an important role in the absorption and metabolism of antipsychotic drugs. Thus, a patient who may absorb a phenothiazine poorly and be refractory as a result, may show a good response to a butyrophenone. The second reason has to do with potency. In general, the more potent antipsychotic agents have a wider effective treatment range. For example, as listed in Table 6-3, the upper dose range of haloperidol is 100 mg/day. An equivalent dose of chlorpromazine would be 5000 mg/day, a dose that few patients could tolerate without experiencing excessive sedation and other troublesome side effects.

The last two guidelines are more general in nature. The first involves the use of polypharmacy. Polypharmacy literally means "many drugs," but the term used clinically refers to the use of two or more antipsychotic drugs concurrently. This practice has never been shown to be more effective than the use of one drug alone in appropriate doses. It also increases the risk of drug interactions and side effects, including tardive dyskinesia. Thus, polypharmacy should be avoided. When a patient does not respond to an antipsychotic agent, the dose of that drug should be increased or the patient should be switched to another drug.

The final guideline concerns the use of antiparkinsonian agents. In the past, these drugs were prescribed prophylactically by many clinicians, and a few recent reports have suggested that these drugs be used routinely to prevent or decrease the severity of extrapyramidal reactions. A good case can be made, however for *not* prescribing these drugs routinely. First, they have not been found to be effective in the prevention of extrapyramidal symptoms. Some studies have shown that they lower serum phenothiazine levels. If this is the case, it would be more prudent to decrease the dose of antipsychotic drug rather than add an antiparkinsonian agent. Perhaps most significant is the fact that these drugs may lower the threshold for the development of tardive dyskinesia, as recent research suggests. Thus, these drugs should not be used routinely, but only to treat extrapyramidal symptoms when they occur.

There is one exception to this general principle and that is with the use of long-acting depot fluphenazine preparations (eg, fluphenazine decanoate). Some patients experience acute dystonic reactions following IM injections of these preparations, associated with the rapid increase of serum fluphenazine levels. These patients may need to take an anti-parkinsonian drug regularly for the week following the injection, when the risk of developing an acute dystonic reaction is greatest.

When antiparkinsonian drugs need to be used, they should be used in the lowest effective dose and for as short a period of time as possible. In general, they should be discontinued after no longer than three to four months, as most studies have shown that less than 10% of patients have extrapyramidal symptoms after this time. Table 6-4 lists the more commonly used antiparkinsonian drugs along with the usual daily dose range of each.

Table 6-4
Commonly Used Antiparkinsonian Drugs*

Generic Name	Trade Name	Usual Daily Dose Range (mg/day)
Anticholinergic Agents		
†Benztropine	Cogentin	1–6
†Biperiden	Akineton	2–6
†Diphenhydramine	Benadryl	25–100
Procyclidine	Kemadrin	6–20
Trihexyphenidyl	Artane, Tremin	2–15
Dopamine Agonist		
Amantadine	Symmetrel	100–300

*By permission from Pirodsky DM: *Primer of Clinical Psychopharmacology: A Practical Guide.* Garden City, NY, Medical Examination Publishing Co Inc, 1981.
†Available in IM and IV preparations for acute dystonic reactions.

These agents pose a dual problem in terms of tardive dyskinesia. It is well known that they exacerbate the symptoms of this disorder, and they may also decrease the threshold for its development. Thus, antiparkinsonian drugs may increase both the incidence and severity of tardive dyskinesia. As with the antipsychotic agents, these drugs should be used judiciously and only when indicated.

7 Neuroleptics and Their Long-Term Effects on the Central Nervous System

George E. Crane

Motor abnormalities induced by neuroleptics usually are subdivided into two categories: those that appear early in the course of treatment and are reversible, and those that manifest themselves late and are irreversible. In the former category are included acute dystonias and parkinsonism, while the latter is represented by tardive dyskinesia. The characteristic buccolingual syndrome, its late appearance in the course of drug therapy, its aggravation as the result of drug withdrawal, and its permanence, are thought to be the essential features of tardive dyskinesia. At least this is the impression one gains from the literature and the package inserts of neuroleptic drugs.

Although the buccolingual syndrome is the best known and the most obvious manifestation of tardive dyskinesia, it is by no means the most important one. Oral involvement may be minimal or even absent in the presence of widespread involvement of the motor apparatus. The unmasking of tardive dyskinesia after drug withdrawal occurs only in certain patients and under certain circumstances, and will be discussed later.

The fact that it is not necessary to discontinue the use of neuroleptics in order to demonstrate the presence of dyskinesia is proven by the large number of dyskinetic patients in hospital wards who are receiving chemotherapy, often in large doses. The problem whether tardive dyskinesia is always irreversible has been questioned in recent years. This matter will be debated indefinitely as long as clinicians fail to agree on certain definitions.

As for dystonia and parkinsonism, they are not always early in appearance or necessarily reversible. In view of all this, the traditional classification of drug-induced neurologic disorders and the definition of tardive dyskinesia require many clarifications and revision. The object of this chapter is "permanent neurologic effects," but all known drug-induced side effects of the central nervous system will be briefly reviewed in order to put tardive dyskinesia and other long-lasting conditions in the proper perspective. Table 7-1 lists all effects of neuroleptics on the brain, including disturbance of sleep and central autonomic imbalance. A classification of these effects of neuroleptics should be as comprehensive as possible, and this table is based on previous efforts published elsewhere.[1]

The widely used Abnormal Involuntary Movement Scale (AIMS) (see Appendix II) lists only motor disorders associated with tardive dyskinesia. For acute dystonia, parkinsonism and other side effects, the investigator must rely on instruments that were developed by the NIMH for their multihospital studies. This dual system is not conducive to a clear understanding of the neurotoxic effects of neuroleptics.

Acute Effects

In this category only dystonia, rapid tremor, and parkinsonism can be considered as being extrapyramidal disorders. Akinesia and akathisia are not, strictly speaking, motor disturbances, although they affect the psychomotor activity of the patient. Both conditions appear relatively early in therapy and are reversible, but they recur when the dosage of medication is increased.

Akinesia is characterized by a disinclination to engage in any type of activity and is accompanied by a feeling of emotional detachment. This response to neuroleptics is often misinterpreted as therapeutic in agitated and troublesome patients. A reduction or elimination of all activities may also minimize tardive dyskinesia. Indifference may cause the patient not to report distressing symptoms, like dystonia, hence the importance of including this item in a comprehensive rating instrument of motor abnormalities.

The main complaint of patients with akathisia is a general feeling of

Table 7-1
Effects of Neuroleptics on the Central Nervous System

Acute*
  Sleep disturbance
  Central autonomic effects
  Dystonia
  Tetanus
  Rapid tremor
  Convulsions
  Parkinsonism (acute)
  Akinesia
  Akathisia
Transient*
  Dyskinesia (adult, juvenile)
  Parkinsonism
  Other (ballismus, tics, etc)
Residual*
  Dyskinesia
  Parkinsonism
Asymptomatic*
  Parkinsonism

Latent†
  Parkinsonism
  Dyskinesia
Tardive Dyskinesia†
  Dyskinesia
  Dystonia
Hypotonia†
Encephalopathies†
  Parkinsonism
  Chorea
  Dystonia
  Tics
  Hemiballismus
  Retrocollis
Chronic Brain Syndrome†
  Dementia

*Reversible and/or clinically insignificant.
†Irreversible, usually disabling when severe.

restlessness; the motor hyperactivity is a secondary phenomenon. It is voluntary and serves the purpose of reducing the distressing urge to be in constant motion. Akathisia only superficially resembles tardive dyskinesia, yet many clinicians are unable to make a distinction between the two syndromes. This confusion is at least in part due to instruments that are incomplete and ambiguous.

The manifestations included in the first category of Table 7-1, are largely the result of a massive absorption of a noxious agent, and the sensitive areas of the central nervous system are unable to cope with this situation. Incidentally, most of the disorders of the first category were described as early manifestations of epidemic encephalitis. Neuroleptics seem to interfere with some crucial step in the metabolism of neurotransmitters at the receptor level. As soon as the noxious agent is removed, symptoms disappear promptly. The use of anticholinergics may restore a normal balance, even though the organism continues to be exposed to neuroleptics. Tolerance also develops after a relatively short period of time. All this suggests that no significant changes have occurred in the functions of the various neuronal units affected by chemotherapy.

Transient Effects

Transient neurologic disorders develop after considerable exposure to drugs and subside slowly,[1,2] rarely rapidly, after neuroleptics have been discontinued.[2,3] In the juvenile type, the symptoms become apparent mainly after withdrawal of medication. Engelhardt refers to these as withdrawal emergent.[4] In the adult type, dyskinesias may be observed while the patient is still on drugs, although an exacerbation of symptoms is possible after the discontinuation of chemotherapy. Transient dyskinesias may become permanent when treatment with neuroleptics is reinstituted, a fact that has been known since 1966.[5]

In the category of transient disorders are tremor and other parkinsonian features, which develop after several months of treatment, respond poorly to anticholinergics, and subside slowly after all drugs are withdrawn. Although there is no clear line of demarcation between the first two categories, the distinction between the two types of parkinsonism is useful in terms of the patient's management.

Ballistic movements, tics and chorea, which are usually chronic (see below), in a few instances may subside or greatly decrease like the transient dyskinesias and parkinsonism.

The slow onset and decline of the transient conditions suggest an alteration of receptor reactivity to dopamine. This disturbance seems to be totally or partially reversible, whereas it is permanent or long lasting in the following categories.

Residual Effects

Transient dyskinesia is by definition temporary, but a careful neurologic examination often reveals abnormal motility in the oral region, and in the fingers and toes, even though no drug is administered for weeks or months. The symptoms are usually intermittent and enhanced by stress. Persons who are self-conscious, as many mental patients are, may be quite concerned about these manifestations; those who are of a litigious disposition may resort to legal action. Otherwise, the residual dyskinesias are clinically insignificant and the patient may not even be aware of them. It is not known whether they disappear eventually, but they may change into the permanent type of dyskinesia with the continued use of drugs. Neuroleptics are not necessarily contraindicated in such cases, but any change in symptomatology should be monitored very closely.

Residual Parkinsonism

Residual parkinsonism consists of occasional bursts of tremors, some loss of associated movements, and/or blankness of facial expression. All this may be observed in patients who have a long-term history of chemotherapy, but are no longer on drugs or receive very small amounts of medication that ordinarily do not cause any extrapyramidal symptoms. In a survey carried out by this author in 1974, about a fourth of patients in a continued treatment service had some evidence of parkinsonism, mainly tremor.[6] In most instances, the symptoms were mild and intermittent. Also noticed was rather severe parkinsonism in some patients; but in such cases, the condition should be assigned to one of the following categories.

Asymptomatic Parkinsonism

Some patients, who have been off drugs or on minimal medication for years, develop a severe form of parkinsonism each time treatment is reinstituted or dosage is increased even to moderate levels. A diagnosis of asymptomatic parkinsonism (in the drug-free period) is justified provided there is no evidence from the history that the patient has an idiosyncrasy to neuroleptics and that similar reactions occurred in the early stages of treatment. Patients in this category are at low risk for more serious side effects of a permanent nature, because the clinical picture is sufficiently dramatic to prompt immediate discontinuation of chemotherapy.

Latent Phenomena

One type of symptom is manifest while another is latent. The treatment status determines what type of symptomatology is present. While adequate doses of a neuroleptic are administered, parkinsonism is evident. When doses are reduced or the medication is discontinued, dyskinesia develops and vice versa. The same shift in the clinical picture occurs when anticholinergics are prescribed, albeit with less predictability. This situation occurs only after the patient has been exposed to neuroleptics for a considerable period of time. Acute parkinsonism of the early stages of therapy with neuroleptics subsides spontaneously, or after the withdrawal of drugs without aftereffects. This is understandable, because chemotherapy was not of sufficient duration to permanently alter receptor functions.

Since the early 1960s, it has been reported that tardive dyskinesia is *unmasked* by the withdrawal of medication. It was my observation that this unmasking could be observed only in certain patients, namely those with parkinsonism. A systematic investigation comparing patients with parkinsonism and patients who were asymptomatic confirmed this impression.[7] Persons afflicted by naturally occurring parkinsonism (and possibly those with the drug-induced disorder) develop dyskinesia when treated with levodopa, while normals do not exhibit such effects. This is consistent with my observations with neuroleptics. Since latent dyskinesia is present mainly in patients with parkinsonian features, a systematic program of drug withdrawal, as recommended by Gardos and Cole,[8] among others, should be carried out first on patients exhibiting some evidence of parkinsonism. As for the management of such patients, it is felt they should not receive neuroleptics at all. There are exceptions where parkinsonism is preferable to tardive dyskinesia.

One of my patients was an elderly female who suffered from apnea and cardiac arrest on three different occasions due to aspiration of food. Drugs in small doses produced a severe form of parkinsonism but controlled the dyskinesia of her pharynx. A similar case was reported by Casey and Rabins.[9]

Tardive Dyskinesia

The term implies abnormal movements and their late appearance in the course of treatment with neuroleptics. When the word *persistent* is added, as in certain package inserts of neuroleptics, the implication is that tardive dyskinesia is irreversible. The term tardive dyskinesia is inadequate, because it does not take into consideration postural abnormalities that are quite common. One should refer to them as tardive dystonias to differentiate them from the acute dystonias that develop very early in treatment. Tremors of a parkinsonian type are abnormal movements, which also may appear late in treatment and become permanent. The rapid oscillatory nature of tremors distinguishes them from the slower and more forceful movements we associate with the dyskinesias. However, the typical pillrolling of parkinsonism has many features in common with the hypermotility of tardive dyskinesia. Finally, there are neurologic syndromes, which are late in appearance, incapacitating and irreversible. However, they resemble systemic neurologic diseases and not the tardive dyskinesias and are referred to as encepalopathies or chronic brain syndrome in my classification.

Despite all these conceptual difficulties, the term tardive dyskinesia should not be abandoned at this time. In the first place, it has been in use for 20 years. Second, the syndrome is reasonably typical and, in most instances, easy to identify. It would be surprising if a common bio-chemical defect underlay all manifestations of tardive dyskinesia. But if one is willing to accept this term, it is essential to define its main components, namely: 1) clinical manifestations, 2) time of appearance, and 3) persistence.

1) The clinical manifestations of tardive dyskinesia have been described extensively by many authors since Sigwald made his first report in the late 1950s.[10] Numerous publications refer to them as choreiform. Although chorea may be present, it is not typical. The movements of tardive dyskinesia are more forceful, better organized, and more likely to always affect specific muscular units. As indicated before, tremors are not part of the syndrome although they may be present in some areas of the body. Certain symptoms in the oral region are referred to as the flycatcher's tongue, the bon bon sign, or the rabbit syndrome.[11] In this regard, it is not thought useful to invent special names for clusters of symptoms, because clinicians have a tendency to ignore manifestations that do not deserve such picturesque designations. (The basic features of abnormal motility are essentially the same, the differences being related to the muscles involved and their functions.) Instead, it is my proposal that the tardive dyskinesias be described according to their anatomical location, severity, regularity, etc. Postural disorders should not be overlooked. Dystonias may be observed in the axial musculature or may be the final stage of a series of involuntary movements of the extremities.

2) Most clinicians and investigators agree that tardive dyskinesia becomes manifest after many months, usually two or three years after ex-posure to drugs. Occasionally, symptoms appear in less than six months. However, my feeling is that the diagnosis in such cases is either incorrect or that the drug histories are inaccurate.

3) Persistent tardive dyskinesia is, by definition, irreversible. This has been documented abundantly.[1] It has been known for many years that the symptomatology decreases in severity over the years provided all medication is discontinued. When this improvement is substantial, the

diagnosis should be transient dyskinesia; and when the remaining symptoms are minimal, we are dealing with residual dyskinesia. Consequently, a diagnosis of tardive dyskinesia can only be tentative when it first appears. A year of observation without drugs may be necessary before a definite diagnosis can be made. In summary, the major characteristics of tardive dyskinesia are: 1) fairly typical abnormal motility and/or posturing, 2) appearance after six months of continuous exposure to drugs, and 3) the presence of at least moderate dyskinesia for about one year after the onset of symptoms.

Hypotonia

This may be a major feature of a neuroleptic induced syndrome, but it is often accompanied by dyskinesias. In addition to impaired tone, which can be detected by a routine examination, there is a loss of associated movements in the upper extremities. The arms swing in an exaggerated manner when the patient begins to walk or when he stops suddenly. During normal deambulation, the arms seem to dangle from the shoulders. In this respect, the picture seems to be the opposite of what one finds in parkinsonism. Whether the loss of tone exaggerates dyskinesia is difficult to say. It is not a prerequisite for abnormal motility, since hyperkinesia also occurs when the tone is normal or even increased.

The proposed classification of the various types of parkinsonism and dyskinesias is largely phenomenological, but is also based on pharmacological consideration.[13] There is a short-term aggravation of dyskinesia as the result of drug withdrawal or the administration of anticholinergics; the opposite is true for parkinsonism. The readministration of neuroleptics will decrease dyskinesia and produce parkinsonism. This is particularly striking in the first category referred to in Table 7-1 as latent. In both conditions there is a tendency to improve after several months of drug-free status, an indication that a partial recovery from the hypothetical disorder at the receptor level is still possible. The more chronic the condition, the less likely is a biochemical normalization.

The last two categories, the encephalopathies and the chronic brain syndromes, show little change over time or in response to pharmacological manipulation.

Encephalopathies

In this category are included various neurologic disorders, which resemble the naturally occurring diseases of the central nervous system.

1. Parkinsonism with tremor, bradykinesia, and rigidity can be observed in a sizeable percentage of elderly persons, who received chemotherapy but are no longer receiving drugs. Since parkinsonism is a fairly common disease after the age of 50 and its prevalence is likely to be higher in a psychiatric hospital than in the general population, assuming an iatrogenic cause is not always justified. Probably the group of parkinsonian patients one sees in a chronic ward is heterogeneous with regard to etiology. Perhaps neuroleptic drugs aggravate or precipitate the condition in predisposed individuals.

2. Chorea predominates in certain patients. In the early 1960s, patients with this syndrome were diagnosed as having Huntington's disease. As a rule, symptoms characteristic of tardive dyskinesia are also in evidence. This, plus the absence of chorea in the family, facilitate the diagnosis.

3. Chronic dystonia is another drug-induced encephalopathy. It may be diffuse, in which case it resembles dystonia musculorum deformans. When localized in the neck, it is torticollis. The sterno-cleido-mastoid muscles may be conspicuously hypertrophic.

4. Tics are probably the most common drug-induced encephalopathies. This category includes bizarre semi-purposeful and complex activities, peculiar vocalizations, etc (see also Chapters 1 and 10).

5. Other encephalopathies are ballismus, retrocollis, and many conditions resembling degenerative diseases of the brain.

All disorders of this type are disabling and do not show a tendency to improve with the passage of time. Patients afflicted by these encephalopathies often come to the attention of neurologists who have little familiarity with drug-induced neurologic side effects. The specialist in neurology or psychiatry finds it difficult to attribute complications of this type to chemotherapy, because the presenting symptoms are inconsistent with those traditionally described for tardive dyskinesia. The ordinary physician is very reluctant to make a diagnosis of an iatrogenic nature, unless he has absolute proof that he is not in error. The standards for noniatrogenic diagnoses are much less rigorous. My position is that all neurologic syndromes developing in the course of intensive drug therapy should be attributed to neuroleptics. The burden is upon the physician to prove that there is a different etiology. This he can do by obtaining a careful history of the onset and sequence of symptoms, by investigating the patient's hereditary background, by ordering appropriate laboratory procedures and by ruling out vascular and neoplastic diseases.

Chronic Brain Syndromes

The encephalopathies are not infrequent and probably grossly underreported. On the other hand, chronic brain syndromes with dementia are extremely rare. From time to time, the literature describes severe loss of higher mental functions due to a neuroleptic.[1] In such cases, the phenothiazine or the butyrophenone may have been prescribed in combination with other agents known to adversely affect the central nervous system. Cohen and Cohen[13] reported severe impairment of the brain in four patients who had received haloperidol plus lithium carbonate. Two patients became irreversibly demented, while the other two recovered only partially. The risk of such catastrophic sequelae is probably not very great. The fact that successful suicide from massive doses of neuroleptics is exceptional seems to confirm this.

Combinations of the manifestations of the various categories of side effects are rather common. Tremors are particularly frequent regardless of the main syndrome and the patient's drug status. An inability to maintain a proper balance between axial segments (dystonia) is seldom observed in the absence of dyskinesias.

Psychic Effects

The question has been asked by many concerned psychiatrists whether neuroleptics aggravate preexisting psychoses or produce new psychological aberrations. Depression from phenothiazines has been reported from time to time. Whether it is caused by neuroleptics is questionable, and at any event, it seems transitory. Occasionally, letters have been received from patients (and from lawyers) claiming all kinds of mental problems that developed after drug therapy often of short duration. Judging from the content of these letters, it is my belief that the alleged difficulties are part of the mental disease for which the drug was prescribed.

There is good reason, however, to be concerned about the long-term effects of chemotherapy on psychoses, particularly schizophrenia. The fact that neuroleptics are beneficial for psychoses does not rule out the possibility that they are injurious in the long run. The progress of schizophrenia to a defect state or severe mental deterioration is a slow process. It must be measured in decades rather than years. Longitudinal studies of 20- or 30-years' duration have not been made on schizophrenics since drugs were introduced in psychiatry.

On theoretical grounds, neuroleptics could accelerate or deepen schizophrenic deterioration. If it is true that an excessive amount of dopamine action at the receptor level plays an important role in the pathogenesis of schizophrenia, the long-term administration of neuroleptics could be very harmful. Phenothiazines and related drugs seem to increase receptor reactivity in the basal ganglia, hence tardive dyskinesia. The same pathological changes may occur in the limbic system or other areas concerned with higher mental functions. A sizeable proportion of schizophrenic patients not only fails to improve but deteriorates mentally despite the use of drugs. Is this unfavorable outcome of the disease the result of drug therapy or is it the terminal state of a malignant form of schizophrenia? The problem is of sufficient importance to deserve an investigation (see Chapter 9).[14]

A representative sample of schizophrenics with long-term hospitalization was studied by this author and mental deterioration was assessed by means of a rating scale designed for this purpose. Data were collected in 1974–1975, or 20 years after neuroleptics were introduced on a large scale in most state hospital systems. The sample consisted of 124 patients with schizophrenia, who had been hospitalized continuously since 1955 and had received the benefit of chemotherapy for most of the duration of their illness. Severe mental deterioration, which could also be called dementia, was evident in about 20% of the sample (17% to 24%, depending on the duration of illness). A large number of studies on chronic schizophrenia were carried out by Kraepelin, Bleuler and their successors in the prepsychopharmacological era. Only two were found that were sufficiently detailed to permit comparisons with my findings.[15,16] According to these two studies, the prevalence of severe deterioration in schizophrenia was twice as large as in my sample. Assuming these comparisons are valid, neuroleptics seem to protect the patient from severe deterioration. At least they do not seem to have an untoward effect on its course.

Another approach is to test the hypothesis that tardive dyskinesia is more prevalent in patients with advanced deterioration than in those less affected by the schizophrenic process. A sample of 234 patients was available for this analysis. Tardive dyskinesia was, indeed, more prevalent in the sicker patients but the difference was not statistically significant. When, on the other hand, the analysis was carried out on a subsample of extremely deteriorated patients, the prevalence of tardive dyskinesia was much higher than in the less mentally impaired schizophrenics. The former may have been exposed to a larger amount of medication, but it is also conceivable that a small minority of schizophrenic patients is very vulnerable to the neurologic and psychic effects of neuroleptic agents.

In conclusion, there is no clear evidence that neuroleptics have a catastrophic effect on the course of schizophrenia. The possible exception is a small, highly susceptible subgroup of schizophrenics who also develop tardive dyskinesia.

Types of Neurologic Disorders and Predisposing Factors

Age and drug exposure generally are related to adverse responses to neuroleptics. The role played by sex and preexisting brain damage is still a matter of controversy. Acute dystonia is more likely to occur in youngsters, while older people are more prone to parkinsonism. In juveniles, transient dyskinesia is almost exclusively limited to the limbs; while in adults, the buccolingual syndrome is at least as common as the abnormal motility of the extremities. A pronounced oral syndrome with sweeping movements of the tongue is probably more common in the elderly. The same applies to violent ballistic movements. Retrocollis with rigidity of the neck was reported only in the very old.[17] The older the patient, the greater the risk of complications, ie, ulcerations of the mouth, dysphagia, and accidents from falls. Encephalopathies, particularly chorea and dystonia, may occur at all ages, but appear to be more common in young adults.

As for drug status, there is considerable evidence that exposure to high doses of powerful neuroleptics is responsible for tardive dyskinesia.[1] The continued use of neuroleptics in patients with transient dyskinesia will eventually lead to permanent dyskinesia. Current drug status plays a crucial role in residual and latent disorders in that the administration of neuroleptics will reveal parkinsonism, while the withdrawal of such agents will uncover dyskinesias. One would expect the encephalopathies to be the result of above average doses, but there have been two known cases where a disabling disorder developed after the administration of neuroleptics in less than average doses. In such cases, an idiosyncratic factor plays a major role.

Therapeutic Considerations

Since the psychiatric community accepted the fact that tardive dyskinesia is a major problem in clinical psychopharmacology, clinicians and pharmacologists have endeavored to find an effective treatment for this disorder. A dozen or more agents have been screened for this purpose. The methodologies and the results of these efforts have been at best dubious, but the recent clinical investigations with choline and lecithin seem to hold some promise (see Chapter 13). Despite the difficulty in finding an effective treatment for tardive dyskinesia, efforts should continue and should be intensified. There are tens of thousands of patients who are incapacitated by tardive dyskinesia and related neurologic disorders. Most of these patients are not likely to improve without a therapeutic intervention. The use of antidotes is no substitute for prevention (see Chapter 14).

This is not to suggest that persistent neurologic side effects can be eliminated completely. Even a cautious and individualized use of drugs has its risks. Some patients require rather large doses of neuroleptics in order to achieve some semblance of mental balance; others may need only average doses, but are highly vulnerable to drug toxicity. Thus, permanent neurologic impairment may be unavoidable in a small percentage of the population treated with chemotherapy. At present, some 50% of patients on long-term drug therapy shows evidence of long-lasting neurotoxicity. This high prevalence of adverse effects and the fact that it is still ignored in many institutions have no precedent in the history of modern medicine.

REFERENCES

1. Crane GE: Tardive dyskinesia and related neurologic disorders, in Iversen LL, Iversen SD, Snyder, SH (eds): *Handbook of Psychopharmacology,* vol X. New York, Plenum Press, 1978.

2. Quitkin F, Rifkin A, Gochfeld L, et al: Tardive dyskinesia: Are first signs reversible? *Am J Psychiatry* 134:84–87, 1977.

3. Crane GE: Rapid reversal of tardive dyskinesia. *Am J Psychiatry* 130:1159, 1973.

4. Polizos, P, Engelhardt D, Hoffman SP: CNS consequences of psychotropic drug withdrawal in schizophrenic children. *Psychopharmacol Bull* 9:34–35, 1973.

5. Schmidt WR, Jarcho LW: Persistent dyskinesias following phenothiazine therapy. *Arch Neurol* 14:369–377, 1966.

6. Crane GE: Factors predisposing to drug-induced neurologic effects, in Forrest I, Carr CJ, Usdin E (eds): *Advances in Biochemical Psychopharmacology. Phenothiazines and Structurally Related Drugs,* vol IX. New York, Raven Press, 1974, pp 269–279.

7. Crane GE: Pseudo-parkinsonism and tardive dyskinesia. *Arch Neurol* 27:426–430, 1972.

8. Gardos G, Cole JO: Maintenance antipsychotic therapy. Is the cure worse than the disease? *Am J Psychiatry* 133:32–36, 1976.

9. Casey DE, Rabins P: Tardive dyskinesia as a life threatening illness. *Am J Psychiatry* 135:486–487, 1978.

10. Sigwald J, Bouttier D, Raymondeaud C, et al: Quatre cas de dyskinesie facio-bucco-linguo-masticatrice a evolution prolongeé secondaire a un traitment par les neuroleptiques. *Rev Neurol* 100:751–755, 1959.

11. Gardos G, Cole JO, LaBrie R, et al: The assessment of tardive dyskinesia. *Arch Gen Psychiatry* 34:1206–1212, 1977.

12. Crane GE: A classification of the neurologic effects of neuroleptic drugs (In press).

13. Cohen WJ, Cohen NE: Lithium carbonate and haloperidol and irreversible brain damage. *JAMA* 230:1283–1287, 1974.

14. Crane GE: Schizophrenic deterioration and drug use. Presented at American Psychiatric Association Annual Meeting, Atlanta, Georgia, May 1978.

15. Freyhan FA: Course and outcome in schizophrenia. *Am J Psychiatry* 112:161–169, 1955.

16. Rennie TAC: Follow-up study of 500 patients with schizophrenia admitted to a hospital 1913 to 1920. *Arch Neurol Psychiatr* 42:877–891, 1939.

17. Harenko A: Retrocollis as an irreversible late complication of neuroleptic medication. *Acta Neurol Scand* 43(suppl 31):145–146, 1967.

8 Clinical Management of Tardive Dyskinesia

Daniel E. Casey
Jes Gerlach

Tardive dyskinesia, a neurological syndrome of involuntary, repetitive, and purposeless movements in the orofacial, limb, and truncal musculature, is associated with the prolonged use of neuroleptic medication. The disturbing trend of increasing prevalence rates, perhaps as high as 20% to 40%, poses a critical problem for maintenance drug treatment of chronic schizophrenia. As the neuroleptic medications are clearly efficacious for many patients, the dilemma is that with continued drug treatment tardive dyskinesia may develop, but without medications the psychosis may worsen. This situation is further complicated by the fact that prior to the onset of symptoms, we cannot predict who is at risk to develop this potentially irreversible neurological syndrome. Though neuroleptic drugs and increasing age are consistently associated with the development of tardive dyskinesia, other demographic variables have not clarified our understanding of the potential vulnerability of the individual patient to develop tardive dyskinesia. Additionally, there is a paucity of information about the natural history of tardive dyskinesia.

This chapter will outline a rational treatment strategy for preventing or managing tardive dyskinesia and also review pharmacological approaches to this syndrome. Though not all cases of tardive dyskinesia can be prevented, early recognition and a well-planned method for managing symptoms are essential because there is no safe and satisfactory treatment. By following these guidelines, it will be possible to minimize the risks and maximize the benefits of neuroleptic treatment.

EVALUATION AND DIAGNOSIS

Epidemiology

Factors predisposing to tardive dyskinesia have been widely studied, but the results are inconsistent. Prevalence rates varied greatly in past studies, from 0.5% to 56%,[1,2] undoubtedly reflecting such variables as criteria for diagnosis and the population of patients studied. Current investigations report that tardive dyskinesia occurs in 20% to 40% of patients maintained on chronic neuroleptic treatment, and that the prevalence increases with advanced age.[3-7] Early reports noted tardive dyskinesia occurred more often in females than in males, but recent studies show a complex interaction between age, sex, and prevalence of tardive dyskinesia. These recent figures apply to both inpatient and outpatient studies, as there are now many chronic schizophrenic patients maintained on neuroleptics in outpatient clinics (see also Chapters 3 and 4).

Clinical Description

The first essential step in managing tardive dyskinesia is to consider the diagnosis. It is important to diagnose tardive dyskinesia early because detection may lead to treatment strategies aimed at preventing further development of the syndrome.[8,9] In addition, distinguishing tardive dyskinesia from syndromes that produce similar clinical pictures may lead to identifying other medical illnesses and movement disorders (see Chapters 1, 5, 10, and 11).

The syndrome of tardive dyskinesia is diagnosed on the basis of a thorough evaluation of drug history, family history, time course of symptoms, demographic and epidemiologic evidence, and a complete physical, neurological, and psychiatric examination. Whereas laboratory tests will help diagnose some hereditary and medical illnesses that produce involuntary movement disorders, there are no laboratory tests for diagnosing tardive dyskinesia. Therefore, the basis of preventing and managing tardive dyskinesia depends on a thorough clinical data base.

Tardive dyskinesia is characterized by involuntary, repetitive, irregular, and purposeless hyperkinetic movements. These symptoms are an admixture of choreic, athetotic, myoclonic, and dystonic features. Abnormal movements in the mouth, tongue, and facial regions are most commonly found.[10] These symptoms usually have an insidious onset with minimal movements that slowly progress to more obvious tongue protrusion, puckering, pursing and smacking of the lips, puffing of the cheeks, or various combinations of jaw movements that resemble chewing. Other facial muscles can be involved, causing rapid eye blinking, blepharospasm, and brow movements.[1,11] Axial musculature can also be affected, producing symptoms of forward and backward pelvic thrusting or continuous rotatory hip motions. Both upper and lower extremities can have a combination of irregular choreic and athetotic movements. Occasionally, the hand and fingers move in a repetitive pattern resembling the playing of an invisible piano or guitar. Rarely, tardive dyskinesia affects the respiratory pattern so that patients make grunting noises and have irregular rates of breathing.[12,13]

Differential Diagnosis

Tardive dyskinesia must be distinguished from the other neuroleptic-induced movement disorders. Acute dystonia most often occurs in young adult males during the first few days of neuroleptic treatment or after a large increase in drug dosage. There is seldom difficulty separating this disorder from tardive dyskinesia, though it is worthwhile restating that persisting dystonic symptoms can be part of the tardive dyskinesia syndrome, especially in children and young adults.[14-16] Akathisia is a subjective feeling of restlessness that may have motor system manifestations of an inability to sit still, tapping of the feet, rapid crossing and uncrossing of the legs, and continuous motion of the trunk. These movements sometimes appear bizarre and can be misdiagnosed as a psychotic exacerbation or tardive dyskinesia.[17] Neuroleptic-induced parkinsonism (tremor, rigidity, and bradykinesia) usually is easily distinguished from tardive dyskinesia. Though the coexistence of tardive dyskinesia and other acute neuroleptic-induced movement disorders is infrequently written about, these dyskinesias may occur in the same patient and can be distinguished by a careful examination.

The rabbit syndrome is characterized by twitching in the lips and perioral area.[18] It is distinguished from tardive dyskinesia by the rapid rhythmical frequency of tremor, localization in the mouth area, and improvement with anticholinergics.[19]

Initial hyperkinesia describes a seldom reported and incompletely understood syndrome that resembles tardive dyskinesia. The symptoms can be difficult to distinguish from tardive dyskinesia because they are clinically similar but may be more stereotyped than tardive dyskinesia.[20] Increased cholinergic influences aggravate the symptoms, which are reversed by anticholinergics, or resolve when neuroleptics are discontinued.[21-25] Although this syndrome is infrequently described, it probably occurs more commonly than is recognized, and emphasizes the point that more than one mechanism may be involved in the etiology of hyperkinetic movement disorders (see also Chapters 3 and 14).

Involuntary dyskinesias also occur with other drug therapies. Levodopa-induced dyskinesias very closely resemble tardive dyskinesia.[26] The anticonvulsants phenytoin, ethosuximide, and carbamazepine can produce or aggravate hyperkinetic dyskinesias that resolve when the drugs are discontinued.[27,28] Choreic movements, as well as stereotyped behavior called "punding," occur in conjunction with sustained amphetamine abuse, and resolve when the stimulants are discontinued.[29] Oral contraceptives may produce temporary choreic symptoms,[30] and long-term antihistamine use has been associated with rare cases of persisting symptoms that resemble tardive dyskinesia.[31] Chloroquine can also produce acute hyperkinetic dyskinesias.[32]

The hereditary neurodegenerative diseases of Huntington's chorea and Wilson's disease (hepatolenticular degeneration) may initially present with signs that resemble tardive dyskinesia, but the later presentations of these syndromes usually are distinguishable by clinical signs, laboratory tests, or the family history. Hyperkinetic movement disorders may be part of the overall constellation of symptoms that occur in endocrine disturbances and general medical illnesses. Hyperthyroidism, hypoparathyroidism, chorea in pregnancy (chorea gravidarum), immune diseases, ie, systemic lupus erythematosus and Henoch-Schonlein's purpura, and postencephalitic syndromes can all be associated with hyperkinetic involuntary mouth movements that resemble tardive dyskinesia.[9]

Although the emphasis thus far has focused on the relationship between hyperkinetic movement disorders and drugs or distinct illnesses, historical perspective reminds us that dyskinesias were associated with, or occurred independently of psychosis prior to the current era of drug therapy. Differing opinions about the association of the psychoses and hyperkinesias can be traced to the original works of Kraepelin and Bleuler. "Athetoid ataxia" was the term used by Kraepelin to describe choreic movements in the face and limbs of chronically institutionalized schizophrenics.[33] On the other hand, Bleuler believed that chorea was associated with organic, not psychologic disease, and attributed this difference in findings to the problem of varying definitions of terms.[34]

More recent investigations have suggested that the high incidence of choreoathetoid disorders described in psychiatric patients in earlier articles overinclusively considered organic neurological diseases.[1,35,36]

A group of phenomenologically similar syndromes of idiopathic hyperkinetic movements in the face, limbs, or trunk can occur in older patients who have never received medications and who do not have psychiatric disorders. These syndromes have been termed "spontaneous orofacial dyskinesia,"[37,38] "spontaneous buccolinguo-facial dyskinesia,"[39] and "blepharospasm-oromandibular dystonia syndrome," also named Brueghel's syndrome or Meige's syndrome.[40-43] These symptoms develop insidiously in patients over 40 years old and usually involve the orofacial region, but may include the limbs and trunk.

Tourette's syndrome of chronic multiple tics and vocalizations differs from tardive dyskinesia by its onset in childhood and the pattern of waxing and waning symptoms. These should be distinguished from simple tics that have persisted throughout life[44] (see Chapter 10).

It is important to reemphasize that the term "tardive dyskinesia" should be reserved for the syndrome of involuntary hyperkinetic movements associated with long-term neuroleptic treatment. Other movement disorders, which are idiopathic, hereditary, involve medical illnesses, or result from other drugs, are not properly termed "tardive dyskinesia" and should be classified separately.

MANAGEMENT

The basic assumptions underlying recommendations for preventing and managing tardive dyskinesia can also be reframed in terms of improving the quality of care for schizophrenia. The elements of an improved treatment plan include: 1) assessment of medication requirements and benefits; 2) use of the appropriate lowest effective dose of neuroleptic treatment; 3) judicious use of anticholinergic drugs; 4) trial periods without neuroleptics; 5) regular reevaluations; and 6) information about the risks of treatment and no treatment.

Medication Requirements and Benefits

Managing patients with tardive dyskinesia, as well as patients taking neuroleptics but not showing dyskinetic symptoms, requires periodic reassessment of the current need for continued neuroleptic treatment. A review of the practice of maintaining neuroleptic medications in outpatients suffering from chronic schizophrenia concluded that approximately 50% of the patients maintained on neuroleptic medications do not relapse when their medicines are discontinued.[45] This implies that half of the patients may be taking more medicine than is necessary. On the other hand, it also implies that if medicines were discontinued in all patients, half of them would be exposed to a potential psychotic exacerbation. This conclusion has been corroborated in additional reviews comparing the protection against relapse by maintenance neuroleptic treatment vs placebo.[5,46] It is also clear that some patients will relapse even while maintained on stable neuroleptic doses. There is no method for determining ahead of time which patients may successfully stop their neuroleptic medications, though the patients' responses to previous drug discontinuation may provide useful information. Deciding to continue or discontinue neuroleptic medications remains a difficult clinical judgment without clearcut guidelines.

Lowest Effective Dose

When the information available suggests that a patient may be able to reduce or discontinue his/her medicines, this should be done. This will prevent the further development of tardive dyskinesia, and may also unmask early signs of tardive dyskinesia that were not evident when the patient was taking neuroleptic drugs. Although rare cases of tardive dyskinesia have been reported after only a few months of neuroleptic treatment,[47,48] most cases occur after treatment has continued for two years or more.[5,49] While some patients develop symptoms during neuroleptic treatment, other patients' symptoms become evident only after the medicines are reduced or discontinued. These may gradually resolve, and have been termed "withdrawal dyskinesia."[50] Early detection, coupled with discontinuation of the neuroleptics, can lead to improvement or complete remission, especially in younger patients.[6] The original psychiatric symptoms may recur, however, and require reinstituting drug therapy.[51] Thus, early diagnosis may reduce the development of irreversible tardive dyskinesia, but produce a dilemma for the patients who have unacceptable side effects from the medicines they need to control psychotic symptoms.

It is important to maintain the patient on the lowest effective dose required to control psychiatric symptoms. This often may be at a lower drug level than the patient is currently taking. A periodic reduction of 10% to 25% in drug dosage will allow the determination of the lowest effective dose. The value of monitoring neuroleptic blood levels, currently in the research and development stages, is a promising but uncharted area. Of particular importance is the question of whether tardive dyskinesia is related to neuroleptic blood levels, as suggested by one recent report.[52] At present, however, treatment decisions must be based on the best clinical judgment, as the neuroleptic drugs have differential effects in patients diagnosed as schizophrenic. While some patients do very well with modest doses, others require substantial daily doses; some benefit very little from neuroleptics; and still others relapse in spite of stable neuroleptic treatment.

Therefore, a single univariate approach of only prescribing the "standard neuroleptic dose" will fail to treat adequately a number of patients. A more broadly based treatment program that emphasizes pharmacological and non-drug approaches is valuable, a conclusion echoed in the thorough reviews of treatment outcomes in long-term management of schizophrenia.[45,53]

The relationship between total neuroleptic dosage, duration of treatment, and tardive dyskinesia is unclear. Though an early report noted this correlation,[54] later studies failed to find an association between total drug intake and tardive dyskinesia.[2,55] More recent studies in primate models of tardive dyskinesia suggest that there is an individual vulnerability to neuroleptics that may make some subjects, through a "reduced buffer capacity," more likely to develop tardive dyskinesia.[20,56-58]

In many instances, continued neuroleptic treatment is necessary in spite of existing tardive dyskinesia because of recurrent psychosis or rarely disabling dyskinesias.[12] Although it is presumed that continued neuroleptic treatment in previously existing tardive dyskinesia will contribute to the further development of this syndrome, there is little research to amplify this question (see below, Drug Treatment, Dopamine Antagonists).

Anticholinergic Drugs

Another important step in managing tardive dyskinesia is to discontinue anticholinergic medicines, when possible. This can frequently be done because the acute extrapyramidal symptoms that initially required anticholinergic treatment often resolve after a few months.[59] There is conflicting correlational evidence both for and against the association of maintenance anticholinergics and the development of tardive dyskinesia,[2,5] but no conclusive consensus. Anticholinergic drugs, however, may temporarily aggravate tardive dyskinesia, once it has developed[20,21,23,60] (see also Chapter 1). Though we do not know if anticholinergics contribute to the pathogenesis of tardive dyskinesia, a drug which is not required and which may be potentially harmful should not be continued.

Trial Periods Without Neuroleptics

The rubric "drug holiday" has been recommended as a way to reduce the risk of tardive dyskinesia, with little evidence either to substantiate or refute this idea. The definition of drug holiday has varied from meaning "never on Sunday" to discontinuing the neuroleptic drugs in all patients for long periods of time. The first definition is not really a drug holiday, but a decrease in the total drug dosage by one-seventh, as the neuroleptics have long pharmacological half-lives. A retrospective investigation reported a higher occurrence of tardive dyskinesia in patients who went on and off neuroleptics than in a comparable group of patients maintained on drug treatment. This raises interesting questions about the role of periodic drug treatment and tardive dyskinesia, but requires further corroboration before the concept of drug discontinuation is concluded to be an etiological factor in tardive dyskinesia.

An advantage of a drug-free interval is that it may uncover mild symptoms of tardive dyskinesia which were previously masked, but which may ultimately be reversible. An additional advantage of periodic drug termination is that patients may be able to function without drug therapy for long periods of time. Psychotic conditions are often characterized by a remitting-relapsing course which may need drug treatment only at specific times. On the other hand, some patients cannot tolerate drug discontinuation, and begin to relapse shortly after reducing or discontinuing medications. This group of patients will probably need to be maintained on a stable level of drug, and at some later time have a trial reduction in drug dosage.

Regular Reexaminations

The long-term management of tardive dyskinesia and chronic mental illnesses requires periodic psychiatric and neurological examinations. It is suggested that at least quarterly evaluations be conducted to augment the initial data base. If possible, more frequent examinations are warranted.

Information About Risks and Benefits

The medical-legal dictum of informed consent is readily finding a place in the recommendations for treating schizophrenia and managing tardive dyskinesia. In theory, this concept says that the patient will be adequately informed about the potential risks of receiving neuroleptic medications, whereas in practice this concept is extremely difficult to implement. There are varied recommendations in the psychiatric literature suggesting that tardive dyskinesia be discussed with patients at different phases of treatment, or that different informed consent documents be prepared for different situations. One recommendation suggests that all patients give informed consent after three months of drug therapy.[61] Other investigators propose that patients who are starting neuroleptic treatment sign informed consent procedures at the beginning of neuroleptic treatment,[62] and patients with tardive dyskinesia sign a separate form at the time the syndrome is diagnosed.[63] A third and more general approach suggests that the clinician inform the patient, as well as a concerned other person, about the risks and benefits of both treatment and no treatment, and that this process be documented in a timely and thoughtful manner consistent with the principles of the doctor-patient relationship.[5,8]

One review of the medical-legal aspects of tardive dyskinesia suggests that the physician is subject to malpractice if he fails to adequately inform the patient about the risks of neuroleptic medications.[64] Though the trend is to recommend informed consent as part of the treatment process, this may become merely a ritual. There are virtually no data to support or refute the basis of this recommendation or to amplify how this process affects compliance with treatment and the long-term outcomes for control of psychoses or development of tardive dyskinesia. If both the medical and legal professions are going to require that informed consent be institutionalized as a part of medical practice, it is important that the patient not be lost in the process (see Chapter 15).

DRUG TREATMENT

In spite of one's best efforts at preventing or minimizing tardive dyskinesia, some patients will need a drug treatment aimed at reducing dyskinetic symptoms. It should be stated at the outset that the currently available pharmacopeia for treating tardive dyskinesia is inadequate, and characterized by questionable efficacy or limiting side effects. The drugs mentioned in the next section include agents aimed at manipulating the dopaminergic, acetylcholinergic, GABAergic, and neuropeptide influences of the basal ganglia. This incomplete list is subject to periodic revision, as many new developments are occurring. In addition, some compounds are restricted to research use only, and are not appropriate for clinical application.

Tardive dyskinesia is hypothesized to develop, at least in part, from dopamine receptor hypersensitivity, perhaps of specific receptor subtypes.[20,65] This may lead to an imbalance between reciprocal dopamine and acetylcholine influences in the nigrostriatal systems. In addition, recent studies in animal models of movement disorders have suggested that neurochemical interrelations in the basal ganglia, which are mediated by GABA and the endorphins, may also play a role in tardive dyskinesia[20,49,58,66] (see also Chapters 1 and 10 to 13).

Dopamine

Dopamine antagonists   The most effective method for suppressing the hyperkinetic symptoms of tardive dyskinesia is to reinstitute a reduction of dopaminergic influences. The effects of different drugs vary, however, depending on a complex interrelationship of 1) striatal antidopaminergic potency; 2) mechanisms of pre- and postsynaptic receptor blockade; 3) catecholamine depletion or synthesis inhibition; and 4) inherent anticholinergic effects. Therefore, it is to be expected that different drugs will not only have many properties in common, but will also have unique characteristics. In any discussion of antidopaminergic drugs for tardive dyskinesia, it is important to raise the caution that treating a syndrome with a group of drugs thought to be the pathophysiological agents causing the syndrome, may temporarily suppress symptoms but then lead to eventual further aggravation.

Recent interest has been shown in reducing dopaminergic influences via presynaptic amine depletion. Reserpine has produced variable effects ranging from nearly complete suppression of tardive dyskinesia to only modest symptomatic improvement with up to 4 mg/day.[1,67,68] If reserpine is used, doses must be started in the antihypertensive range of approximately 0.25 mg/day and gradually increased. Potential side effects of depression, hypotension, diarrhea, and nasal congestion may be encountered as the doses are gradually increased. Other research strategies with the amine depletors have included tetrabenazine[69] and α-methyl-p-tyrosine.[70,71] Although reserpine has only rarely been associated with causing tardive dyskinesia, it should be cautiously considered as a treatment because the caveat holds that it may be reproducing the neurochemical imbalance that is implicated in an animal model of tardive dyskinesia.[72]

Theoretically all the neuroleptics commercially available are capable of temporarily masking tardive dyskinesia. However, whether one particular drug is more capable than another of suppressing tardive dyskinesia is a subject of ongoing research. Haloperidol (Haldol), a low-milligram, high-potency dopamine receptor blocker, strongly reduced tardive dyskinesia,[73,74] though there was a gradual breakthrough of symptoms by the end of four months.[73] Thioridazine (Mellaril), a high-milligram, low-potency dopamine receptor blocker, also reduced tardive dyskinesia, though less than haloperidol.[74] The effects of these neuroleptics in tardive dyskinesia may change in the course of prolonged treatment over many years, however. Though long-term studies of suppressing tardive dyskinesia with neuroleptics or reserpine are limited, we have been able to maintain patients on low doses of neuroleptics for up to four years without aggravating tardive dyskinesia. This observation has also been noted in a larger longitudinal study.[67]

The potential of neuroleptics to induce reversible or irreversible tardive dyskinesia is a related ongoing concern. Many retrospective epidemiological studies have attempted to clarify the relationship between drug type, dosage, and duration of treatment, but the results have been inconsistent. This may not be surprising, however, if the predisposing vulnerability of the individual to develop tardive dyskinesia is of greater importance than varying drug parameters. More valid data addressing this question will come from prospective studies of large groups of patients. A promising direction of research has been the development of a nonhuman primate model of tardive dyskinesia and behavioral hypersensitivity.[56,57,75,76] These investigations in monkeys support the concept that there is an individual predisposition for developing tardive dyskinesia and hypersensitivity that covaries with dose and duration of treatment.

A separate line of investigation has been to evaluate the propensity of specific neuroleptics to affect dopaminergic influences in different brain regions. A prospective study showed that after treatment with haloperidol 5 mg/day the rebound aggravation of tardive dyskinesia was greater than after the initial treatment with thioridazine 250 mg/day, whereas the antipsychotic effect of these two compounds was equal.[74] These results suggest that haloperidol is more potent than thioridazine in its ability to suppress and produce rebound aggravation of tardive dyskinesia. This observation is supported by studies in monkeys in which the exacerbation of irreversible tardive dyskinesia following a single challenge dose of haloperidol was more prolonged than the corresponding response to an equipotent dose of thioridazine.[76] Recent research has also shown that thioridazine may preferentially inhibit dopamine receptors in the limbic system,[77] thus supporting the suggestion that the lower prevalence of extrapyramidal syndromes with thioridazine is not exclusively due to its anticholinergic properties (see also Chapter 11). These experiments were limited to short-term studies, however, and must be extended to long-term trials to more thoroughly evaluate drug differences. Neuroleptic treatment for up to one year in rodents with thioridazine and trifluoperazine (Stelazine) did not show any differences in the ability of these drugs to produce behavioral and biochemical hypersensitivity.[78,79]

Successful suppression of tardive dyskinesia may also involve producing or aggravating parkinsonian symptoms.[74,80] This problem may be partly managed by using the high-milligram, low-potency neuroleptics, ie, thioridazine or chlorpromazine (Thorazine), because they produce fewer acute extrapyramidal symptoms. An interesting new approach evolving from research in Europe is to use selective dopamine receptor blockers of the type-2 dopamine receptor, ie, sulpiride or oxiperomide.[81-83] Sulpiride, a novel neuroleptic of the substituted benzamide class, differs in some respects from the classical neuroleptics. It inhibits apomorphine-induced stereotyped behavior but does not induce pronounced catalepsy, and increases dopamine turnover and prolactin secretion without inhibiting the dopamine-stimulated adenylcyclase.[84] In studies with sulpiride and oxiperomide, tardive dyskinesia scores were significantly suppressed, whereas parkinsonian scores did not significantly change during drug treatment. During the placebo phase, tardive dyskinesia scores returned to baseline level, suggesting that separate mechanisms, at least in part, control the neuroleptic-induced hypokinetic symptoms of parkinsonism and the hyperkinetic symptoms of tardive dyskinesia.

Whether the proposed type-2 dopamine receptor blockers are more or less likely to produce or affect tardive dyskinesia than the classical neuroleptics cannot be concluded from the available data. Though the hypotheses about relationships between different dopamine receptors, pharmacological effects, and various dyskinesias are intriguing, these suggestions are unsubstantiated and must be thoroughly tested in comparative clinical trials and with animal models of tardive dyskinesia. The ultimate goal of psychopharmacological research is to develop an effective antipsychotic drug that is free of neurological and other troublesome side effects.

Dopamine agonists Altering the purported dopamine receptor hypersensitivity underlying tardive dyskinesia has been attempted with drugs that increase available dopamine. This approach reasons that if dopamine receptors have developed increased sensitivity due to receptor blockade, stimulating the receptors with dopamine agonists might "reset" receptor sensitivity to a normal range of function. Recent animal studies have shown that both the biochemical and behavioral signs of dopamine receptor hypersensitivity are decreased following treatment with levodopa,[85,86] but results in clinical trials are inconsistent. The initial and subsequent studies with levodopa (see Chapter 12) reported encouraging results in tardive dyskinesia. However, in elderly patients with irreversible tardive dyskinesia, the reduction in symptoms was small after levodopa + benserazine (Madopar) 600 mg/day (corresponding to 3000 mg/day of levodopa) for four weeks; in patients receiving neuroleptic drugs, Madopar 900 mg/day (corresponding to 4500 mg/day of levodopa) had no effect.[87] This result was confirmed in a subsequent trial with Madopar up to 1600 mg/day (corresponding to 8000 mg/day of levodopa) for eight weeks.[88] In one patient not receiving neuroleptics, only a slight improvement in tardive dyskinesia occurred. No clinically significant effects on tardive dyskinesia were otherwise observed. Four patients experienced undesirable side effects of depression, increased psychosis, or agitation. These limited findings have also been seen when levodopa + carbidopa (Sinemet) has been used to treat blepharospasm.[43]

Direct receptor stimulation with dopamine agonists has also been used in experimental trials for tardive dyskinesia. Apomorphine, a partial dopamine agonist, usually decreased tardive dyskinesia, perhaps through presynaptic mechanisms.[89,90] The ergot dopamine agonists bromocriptine (Parlodel) and CF 25-397 failed to affect tardive dyskinesia.[91] These inconsistent findings with dopamine agonists will require further study to provide additional information about the mechanisms of actions and the clinical effects of dopamine agonists in tardive dyskinesia.

Acetylcholine

Anticholinergics Cholinergic hypofunction is a purported pathophysiological factor underlying tardive dyskinesia, possibly interacting with dopamine receptor hypersensitivity. As discussed above, anticholinergic drugs can aggravate or uncover existing tardive dyskinesia.[21,23,65,70] Anticholinergics, when given in combination with neuroleptics, may markedly reduce the antihyperkinetic effect of neuroleptics on tardive dyskinesia.[74] In a few reports, anticholinergics have reduced rather than aggravated tardive dyskinesia.[21-23] It is not yet clear if there is a subgroup of patients with tardive dyskinesia that may benefit from anticholinergics, or if these infrequently reported cases of improvement with anticholinergics actually represent patients with the seldom recognized syndrome of initial hyperkinesia (described above).

Cholinergic agonists Augmenting a relatively underfunctioning cholinergic system has been a logical experimental approach to treating tardive dyskinesia. Physostigmine, an acetylcholine esterase inhibitor, usually decreased tardive dyskinesia, but may have variable effects[21,23,60,92,93] that are complicated by undesirable effects of sedation, dizziness, nausea, and vomiting. The initial attempts to treat tardive dyskinesia via cholinergic precursor loading were with deanol

(Deaner).[94,95] Though choline blood levels are increased with deanol, the effect of this compound on cholinergic mechanisms is unclear.[96] Later investigations and a review of deanol in movement disorders concluded this drug produces inconsistent results in hyperkinetic dyskinesias.[97] Choline moderately reduced tardive dyskinesia symptoms,[93,98,99] though side effects limit the widespread use of this compound. Lecithin (phosphatidylcholine), like choline, also raises blood choline levels and may[100,101] or may not[102] reduce tardive dyskinesia (see also Chapter 13). Though the idea that the cholinergic system could be modified by precursor loading is theoretically attractive, further research is needed to develop practical, effective, and safe compounds. It is also necessary to clarify the question of whether choline blood levels accurately reflect central nervous system cholinergic processes and provide a mechanism for altering disease states.

GABA

Recent investigations of striatonigral mechanisms suggest that increased GABAergic influences may have an inhibitory effect on dopaminergic function.[103] The GABA agonist muscimol decreased tardive dyskinesia,[104] but this experimental compound has untoward psychotomimetic effects.[105] Gamma-acetylenic-GABA, an irreversible catalytic inhibitor of the degradative enzyme GABA-transaminase, also significantly reduced tardive dyskinesia.[106] Interestingly, this experimental GABA agonist had significantly greater antihyperkinetic effects in patients taking neuroleptic drugs, suggesting that increased GABA influences may reduce tardive dyskinesia by indirect effects on dopaminergic mechanisms.

Sodium valproate (Depakene) may increase brain GABA via GABA-transaminase inhibition, though there is some question whether doses used in the clinic are large enough to affect brain GABA. After the initial positive report of sodium valproate in tardive dyskinesia,[107] less encouraging results have been reported.[108-111] As with gamma-acetylenic GABA, sodium valproate was more effective in suppressing tardive dyskinesia when it was combined with a neuroleptic.[111] Baclofen (Lioresal), a structural analog of GABA, with unclear effects on GABA mechanisms, moderately suppressed tardive dyskinesia[112]; potentiated the neuroleptic antihyperkinetic effects[111,113]; and was substantially less effective in suppressing tardive dyskinesia when not used in combination with neuroleptics.[111]

Benzodiazepines may also act as GABA agonists. Diazepam (Valium) has both reduced[114-116] and aggravated tardive dyskinesia,[117] but further controlled trials are needed to corroborate these reports. Clonazepam (Clonopin), a benzodiazepine that may also affect serotonin, also reduced tardive dyskinesia.[118] More recently, this drug was reported to be as effective as phenobarbital in reducing tardive dyskinesia,[119] and again raises the question of whether the anti-hyperkinetic effects of benzodiazepines in tardive dyskinesia occur primarily through GABAergic mechanisms, via nonspecific sedative effects, or through other processes.

Neuropeptides

The recent identification of endogenous opiate receptors in the central nervous system has stimulated much research into the effects of these neurochemical systems in psychiatric and neurological syndromes. The β-lipotropin hormone,$_{61-91}$(β-LPH$_{61-91}$) compound and its peptide fragments have been found to affect dopamine-mediated mechanisms, and thus may be involved in the pathophysiology of schizophrenia and tardive dyskinesia. Though research with these compounds is entirely at the experimental level, the effects of these neuropeptides on tardive dyskinesia may lead to a greater understanding of involuntary movement disorders, and to the development of clinically useful compounds. Similar to the strategy of investigating the role of other neurotransmitters in clinical trials, the effects of the neuropeptide agonists and antagonists have been studied in tardive dyskinesia.

The met-enkephalin (β-LPH$_{61-65}$) synthetic analog FK 33-824 was compared with the naturally occurring agonist morphine, and the antagonist naloxone (Narcan). FK 33-824 produced only a modest suppression of tardive dyskinesia; even less effect was produced by morphine. The most pronounced decrease in tardive dyskinesia with either drug was seen in patients who were concurrently receiving a high neuroleptic dose.[120] These findings correspond to the effect of the putative GABA agonists discussed earlier, and are consistent with a proposal of indirect influences on dopaminergic mechanisms. Naloxone, an opiate antagonist, had no consistent effect on tardive dyskinesia.[120] Recent reports have shown that the non-opiate β-LPH$_{62-77}$ fragment, des-tyrosine-γ-endorphin (DTγE), also had no effect on tardive dyskinesia.[121,122] The initial results do not suggest a primary role for these specific peptide fragments in the pathophysiology or treatment of tardive dyskinesia. However, this area of drug development is still in the early stages, and new molecular subdivisions of the β-lipotropin hormone will undoubtedly be considered in future tardive dyskinesia research.

Other Drug Trials

Many other medications for tardive dyskinesia have been investigated, varying from controlled trials to individual case reports. Although the initial reports with lithium carbonate were encouraging, later double-blind studies showed minimal or no benefit in patients with long-term severe tardive dyskinesia.[123,124] Lithium offers little promise as a primary treatment for tardive dyskinesia, but is an important drug in the armamentarium for treating affective psychoses. When patients with diagnoses of schizophrenia and tardive dyskinesia also have affective symptoms, an adequate clinical trial with lithium may be able to replace the neuroleptic medication and thus reduce the long-term risks of tardive dyskinesia. Papaverine, a derivative of opium, moderately decreased tardive dyskinesia, perhaps through its weak dopamine antagonist properties.[125] Estrogen also reduced tardive dyskinesia.[126,127] Hydergine, an ergot alkaloid, may reduce tardive dyskinesia.[128] Cyproheptadine (Periactin), a mixed antihistaminic, antiserotoninergic compound, has produced inconsistent results.[129] Tryptophan has not been generally effective in tardive dyskinesia.[114,130] Amantadine (Symmetrel) and methylphenidate (Ritalin) also have inconsistently affected tardive dyskinesia.[131-134] High dose pyridoxine may be effective in moderately suppressing tardive dyskinesia,[135] whereas lower doses were ineffective.[136] Clonidine (Catapres)[137] and propranolol (Inderal)[138] are also under investigation as potential treatments for tardive dyskinesia.

SUMMARY

The pathophysiological mechanisms underlying tardive dyskinesia have been partly clarified through the systematic approach of pharmacological manipulations of putative central nervous system neurotransmitters. Evidence indicates that dopamine is primarily involved in tardive dyskinesia, as drugs which decrease the availability of dopamine consistently suppress hyperkinetic symptoms. The role of dopamine agonists in tardive dyskinesia, however, remains unclear. Further research must clarify and expand the developing evidence of dopamine receptor subtypes, and produce drugs that translate the biochemical differences identified in the laboratory into highly specific agents to be used in the clinic. The formulation of new and unique neuroleptics offers the hope of successfully treating schizophrenia without the liability of producing tardive dyskinesia.

Cholinergic mechanisms play a secondary and incompletely understood role in tardive dyskinesia. Additional research is needed to clarify the effects of prolonged anticholinergic treatment in the etiology of tardive dyskinesia. Developing more effective cholinergic agonists and elucidating the effects of precursor loading on central nervous system cholinergic function may provide new treatment approaches for managing tardive dyskinesia. At the current level of investigation, neither the GABA nor endorphin system seems to play a direct role in the pathophysiology or treatment of tardive dyskinesia. Rather, the effects of these systems may indirectly affect dopaminergic mechanisms. New compounds undoubtedly will be developed and serve as important research tools for expanding our understanding of tardive dyskinesia, other movement disorders, and psychoses.

During the past two and one-half decades, neuroleptic medications have provided a practical and efficacious treatment of acute and chronic psychoses. It is clear, however, that this advancement in clinical psychopharmacology has been at the unanticipated cost of producing the potentially irreversible neurological syndrome of tardive dyskinesia. This tradeoff between risks and benefits now leads to a timely reassessment of the clinical use of neuroleptic medications. The overall ineffectiveness or troublesome side effects of the currently available clinical and research drugs to treat tardive dyskinesia supports the contention that it will be far better to direct efforts toward preventing the syndrome than trying to control tardive dyskinesia once it develops. As we minimize the risks and maximize the benefits of appropriate neuroleptic treatment, tardive dyskinesia will become a less frequent and less disabling consequence of psychopharmacological treatment of psychoses.

ACKNOWLEDGMENTS

We thank Marian K. Karr for expertly preparing the typescript. This work was supported in part by grants from the Veterans Administration Research Career Development program and The Grass Foundation.

REFERENCES

1. Crane GE: Persistent dyskinesia. *Br J Psychiatry* 122:395–405, 1973.

2. Jus A, Pineau R, Lachance R, et al: Epidemiology of tardive dyskinesia. *Dis Nerv Syst* 37:210–214, 257–261, 1976.

3. Asnis GM, Leopold MA, Duvoisin RC, et al: A survey of tardive dyskinesia in psychiatric outpatients. *Am J Psychiatry* 134:1367–1370, 1977.

4. Smith JM, Kucharski LT, Eblen C: An assessment of tardive dyskinesia in schizophrenic outpatients. *Psychopharmacol* 64:99–104, 1979.

5. APA Task Force Report 18. Edited by R. Baldessarini et al. American Psychiatric Association, 1980.

6. Smith JM, Baldessarini RJ: Changes in prevalence, severity and recovery in tardive dyskinesia with age. *Arch Gen Psychiatry* 37:1368-1373, 1980.

7. Jeste DV, Wyatt RJ: Changing epidemiology of tardive dyskinesia: an overview. *Am J Psychiatry* 138:297-309, 1981.

8. Casey DE: Managing tardive dyskinesia. *J Clin Psychiatry* 39:748-753, 1978.

9. Casey DE: The differential diagnosis of tardive dyskinesia. *Acta Psychiatr Scand* (suppl 291)63:71-87, 1981.

10. Uhrbrand L, Faurbye A: Reversible and irreversible dyskinesia after treatment with perphenazine, chlorpromazine, reserpine and electroconvulsive therapy. *Psychopharmacol* 1:408-418, 1960.

11. Stevens JR: Eye blink and schizophrenia: psychosis or tardive dyskinesia? *Am J Psychiatry* 135:223-226, 1978.

12. Casey DE, Rabins P: Tardive dyskinesia as a life-threatening illness. *Am J Psychiatry* 135:486-488, 1978.

13. Weiner WJ, Goetz CG, Nausieda PA, et al: Respiratory dyskinesias, extrapyramidal dysfunction and dyspnea. *Ann Intern Med* 88:327-331, 1978.

14. Polizos P, Engelhardt DM, Hoffman SP: Neurological consequences of psychotropic drug withdrawal in schizophrenic children. *J Autism Child Schizo* 3:247-253, 1973.

15. McAndrew JB, Case Q, Trefert DA: Effects of prolonged phenothiazine intake on psychotic and other hospitalized children. *J Autism Child Schizo* 2:75-91, 1972.

16. McLean P, Casey DE: Tardive dyskinesia in an adolescent. *Am J Psychiatry* 135:969-971, 1978.

17. Van Putten T: The many faces of akathisia. *Compr Psychiatry* 16:43-47, 1975.

18. Villeneuve A: The rabbit syndrome: a peculiar extrapyramidal reaction. *Can Psychiatr Assoc J* 17:69-72, 1972.

19. Sovner R, DiMascio A: The effect of benztropine mesylate in the rabbit syndrome and tardive dyskinesia. *Am J Psychiatry* 134:1301-1302, 1977.

20. Gerlach J: Tardive dyskinesia. *Dan Med Bull* 26:209-245, 1979.

21. Gerlach J, Reisby N, Randrup A: Dopaminergic hypersensitivity and cholinergic hypofunction in the pathophysiology of tardive dyskinesia. *Psychopharmacol* 34:21-35, 1974.

22. Granacher RP, Baldessarini RJ, Cole JO: Deanol for tardive dyskinesia. *N Engl J Med* 292:926-927, 1975.

23. Casey DE, Denney D: Pharmacological characterization of tardive dyskinesia. *Psychopharmacol* 54:1-8, 1977.

24. Glazer WM, Moore DC: The diagnosis of rapid abnormal involuntary movements associated with fluphenazine decanoate. *J Nerv Ment Dis* 168:439-441, 1980.

25. Moore DC, Bowers MB: Identification of a subgroup of tardive dyskinesia patients by pharmacologic probes. *Am J Psychiatry* 137:1202-1205, 1980.

26. Gerlach J: Relationship between tardive dyskinesia, L-dopa-induced hyperkinesia and parkinsonism. *Psychopharmacol* 51:259-263, 1977.

27. Chadwick D, Reynolds EH, Marsden CD: Anticonvulsant-induced dyskinesias: a comparison with dyskinesias induced by neuroleptics. *J Neurol Neurosurg Psychiatry* 39:1210-1218, 1976.

28. DeVeaugh-Geiss J: Aggravation of tardive dyskinesia by phenytoin. *N Engl J Med* 298:457-458, 1978.

29. Rylander G: Psychoses and punding and choreiform syndromes in addiction to central stimulant drugs. *Psychiatr Neurol Neurochirg* 75:203–212, 1972.

30. Nausieda PA, Koller WC, Weiner WJ, et al: Chorea induced by oral contraceptives. *Neurology* 29:1605–1609, 1979.

31. Thach BT, Chase TN, Bosma JF: Oral facial dyskinesia associated with prolonged use of antihistaminic decongestants. *N Engl J Med* 293:486–487, 1975.

32. Osifo NG: Drug-related transient dyskinesias. *Clin Pharmacol Ther* 25:767–771, 1979.

33. Kraepelin E: *Dementia Praecox and Paraphrenia.* Edinburgh, E&S Livingstone, 1919, pp 43–83.

34. Bleuler E: *Dementia Praecox or the Group of Schizophrenias.* New York, International Universities Press, 1950.

35. Mettler FA, Crandall A: Neurologic disorders in psychiatric institutions. *J Nerv Ment Dis* 128:148, 1959.

36. Jones M, Hunter R: Abnormal movements in patients with chronic psychiatric illness, in *Psychotropic Drugs and Dysfunctions of the Basal Ganglia.* U.S. Public Health Service Publication 1938, 1969.

37. Altrocchi PH: Spontaneous oral-facial dyskinesia. *Arch Neurol* 26:506–512, 1972.

38. Pakkenberg H, Fog R: Spontaneous oral dyskinesia. *Arch Neurol* 31:352–353, 1974.

39. Delwaide PJ, Desseilles M: Spontaneous buccolinguofacial dyskinesia in the elderly. *Acta Neurol Scand* 56:256–262, 1977.

40. Meige H: Les convulsions de la face, une forme clinique de convulsion faciale, bilaterale et mediane. *Revue Neurologique* 20:437, 1910.

41. Marsden CD: Blepharospasm-oromandibular dystonia syndrome (Brueghel's syndrome). *J Neurol Neurosurg Psychiatry* 39:1204–1209, 1976.

42. Tolosa E, Lai C: Meige's disease: striatal dopaminergic preponderance. *Neurology* 29:1126–1130, 1979.

43. Casey DE: Pharmacology of blepharospasm-oromandibular dystonia syndrome. *Neurology* 30:690–695, 1980.

44. Sweet RD, Solomon GE, Wayne H, et al: Neurological features of Gilles de la Tourette's syndrome. *J Neurol Neurosurg Psychiatry* 36:1–9, 1973.

45. Gardos G, Cole JO: Maintenance antipsychotic therapy: Is the cure worse than the disease? *Am J Psychiatry* 133:32–36, 1976.

46. Davis JM: Overview: Maintenance therapy in psychiatry: I. Schizophrenia. *Am J Psychiatry* 132:1237–1245, 1975.

47. Faurbye A, Rasch PJ, Bender Peterson P, et al: Neurologic symptoms in the pharmacotherapy of psychoses. *Acta Psychiatr Scand* 40:10–26, 1964.

48. Chouinard G, Jones BD: Early onset of tardive dyskinesia: Case report. *Am J Psychiatry* 136:1323–1324, 1979.

49. Tarsy D, Baldessarini RJ: The tardive dyskinesia syndrome, in Klawans HL (ed): *Clinical Neuropharmacology,* vol 1. New York, Raven Press, 1976, pp 29–61.

50. Gardos G, Cole JO, Tarsy D: Withdrawal syndromes associated with antipsychotic drugs. *Am J Psychiatry* 135:1321–1324, 1978.

51. Quitkin F, Rifkin A, Gochfeld L, et al: Tardive dyskinesia: Are first signs reversible? *Am J Psychiatry* 134:84–87, 1977.

52. Jeste DV, Rosenblatt JE, Wagner RL, et al: High serum neuroleptic levels in tardive dyskinesia? *N Engl J Med* 301:1184, 1979.

53. May PRA: Rational treatment for an irrational disorder: What does

the schizophrenic patient need? *Am J Psychiatry* 133:1008–1012, 1976.

54. Crane GE, Smeets RA: Tardive dyskinesia and drug therapy in geriatric patients. *Arch Gen Psychiatry* 30:341–343, 1974.

55. Simpson GM, Varga E, Lee HJ, et al: Tardive dyskinesia and psychotropic drug history. *Psychopharmacol* 58:117–124, 1978.

56. Gunne LM, Barany S: Haloperidol-induced tardive dyskinesia in monkeys. *Psychopharmacol* 50:237–240, 1976.

57. Casey DE, Gerlach J, Christensson E: Behavioral aspects of dopamine receptor hypersensitivity in primates. *Prog Neuro-Psychopharmacol* (suppl)110: 101, 1980.

58. Casey DE, Gerlach J, Korsgaard S: Clinical pharmacological approaches to evaluating tardive dyskinesia, in Usdin E, Dahl S, Gram LF, et al (eds): *Clinical Pharmacology in Psychiatry*. New York, Macmillan, 1981 (In press).

59. Orlov P, Kasparian G, DiMascio A, et al: Withdrawal of antiparkinson drugs. *Arch Gen Psychiatry* 25:410–412, 1971.

60. Klawans HL, Rubovits R: Effect of cholinergic and anticholinergic agents on tardive dyskinesia. *J Neurol Neurosurg Psychiatry* 37:941–947, 1974.

61. Ayd FJ: Ethical and legal dilemmas posed by tardive dyskinesia. *Int Drug Ther Newsletter* 12:29–36, 1977.

62. DeVeaugh-Geiss J: Informed consent for neuroleptic therapy. *Am J Psychiatry* 136:959–962, 1979.

63. Sovner R, DiMascio A, Berkowitz D, et al: Tardive dyskinesia and informed consent. *Psychosomatics* 19:172–177, 1978.

64. Slovenko R: On the legal aspects of tardive dyskinesia. *J Psychiatry & Law J* 295–331, 1979

65. Klawans HL: The pharmacology of tardive dyskinesia. *Am J Psychiatry* 130:82–86, 1973.

66. Mackay AVP, Sheppard GP: Pharmacotherapeutic trials in tardive dyskinesia. *Br J Psychiatry* 135:489–499, 1979.

67. Jus A, Jus K, Fontaine P: Long-term treatment of tardive dyskinesia. *J Clin Psychiatry* 40:72–77, 1979.

68. Sato S, Daly R, Peters H: Reserpine therapy of phenothiazine-induced dyskinesia. *Dis Nerv Syst* 32:680–685, 1971.

69. Kazamatsuri H, Chien C, Cole JO: The treatment of tardive dyskinesia. I. Clinical efficacy of a dopamine-depleting agent, tetrabenazine. *Arch Gen Psychiatry* 27:95–99, 1972.

70. Gerlach J, Thorsen K: The movement pattern of oral tardive dyskinesia in relation to anticholinergic and antidopaminergic treatment. *Int Pharmacopsychiatry* 11:1–7, 1976.

71. Magelund G, Gerlach J, Casey DE: Neuroleptic-potentiating effect of α-methyl-p-tyrosine compared with haloperidol and placebo in a double-blind crossover trial. *Acta Psychiatr Scand* 60:185–189, 1979.

72. Tarsy D, Baldessarini RJ: Behavioral supersensitivity to apomorphine following chronic treatment with drugs which interfere with the synaptic function of catecholamines. *Neuropharmacol* 13:927–940, 1974.

73. Kazamatsuri H, Chien C, Cole JO: The treatment of tardive dyskinesia. II. Short-term efficacy of dopamine-blocking agents haloperidol and thiopropazate. *Arch Gen Psychiatry* 27:100–103, 1972.

74. Gerlach J, Simmelsgaard H: Tardive dyskinesia during and following treatment with haloperidol, haloperidol + biperiden, thioridazine, and clozapine. *Psychopharmacol* 59:105–112, 1978.

75. Carlson KR, Eibergen RD: Susceptibility to amphetamine-elicited dyskinesias following chronic methadone treatment in monkeys. *Ann NY Acad Sci* 281:336–349, 1976.

76. Gunne LM, Barany S: A monitoring test for the liability of neuroleptic drugs to induce tardive dyskinesia. *Psychopharmacol* 63:195–198, 1979.

77. Borison RL, Havdala HS, Diamond BI: Intralimbic administration of antipsychotic drugs. *Proc Ann Am Psychiatric Assoc Meet* 41:80–81, 1980.

78. Clow A, Jenner P, Marsden CD: Changes in dopamine-mediated behavior during one year's neuroleptic administration. *Eur J Pharmacol* 57:365–375, 1979.

79. Clow A, Theodorou A, Jenner P, et al: Changes in rat striatal dopamine turnover and receptor activity during one year's neuroleptic administration. *Eur J Pharmacol* 63:135–144, 1980.

80. Claveria LE, Teychenne PF, Calne DB: Tardive dyskinesia treated with pimozide. *J Neurol Sci* 24:393–401, 1975.

81. Casey DE, Gerlach J, Simmelsgaard H: Sulpiride in tardive dyskinesia. *Psychopharmacol* 66:73–77, 1979.

82. Casey DE, Gerlach J: Oxiperomide in tardive dyskinesia. *J Neurol Neurosurg Psychiatry* 43:264–267, 1980.

83. Häggström JE: Sulpiride in tardive dyskinesia. *Curr Ther Res* 27:164–169, 1980.

84. Jenner P, Clow A, Reavill C, et al: A behavioral and biochemical comparison of dopamine receptor blockade produced by haloperidol with that produced by substituted benzamide drugs. *Life Sci* 23:545–550, 1978.

85. Ezrin-Waters C, Seeman P: L-dopa reversal of hyperdopaminergic behavior. *Life Sci* 22:1027–1032, 1978.

86. Friedhoff AJ, Rosengarten H, Bonnet K: Receptor-cell sensitivity modification (RSM) as a model for pathogenesis and treatment of tardive dyskinesia, in Fann WE, Smith RC, Davis JM, et al (eds): *Tardive Dyskinesia Research and Treatment.* New York, SP Medical and Scientific Books, 1980, pp 139–143.

87. Gerlach J: Pathophysiological aspects of reversible and irreversible tardive dyskinesia, in Obiols J, Ballus C, Monclus G, et al (eds): *Biological Psychiatry Today,* vol A. New York, Elsevier, 1979, pp 653–657.

88. Bjørndal N, Casey DE, Gerlach J, et al: The effect of levodopa in tardive dyskinesia, in Usdin E, Eckert H, Forrest I (eds): *Phenothiazines and Structurally Related Drugs: Basic and Clinical Studies.* New York, Elsevier, 1980, pp 321–324.

89. Carroll BJ, Curtis GC, Kokmen E: Paradoxical response to dopamine agonists in tardive dyskinesia. *Am J Psychiatry* 134:785–789, 1977.

90. Smith RC, Tamminga C, Davis JM: Effect of apomorphine on schizophrenic symptoms. *J Neural Transm* 40:171–176, 1977.

91. Tamminga CA, Chase TN: Bromocriptine and CF 25-397 in the treatment of tardive dyskinesia. *Arch Neurol* 37:204–205, 1980.

92. Tarsy D, Leopold N, Sax DS: Physostigmine in choreiform movement disorders. *Neurology* 24:28–33, 1974.

93. Davis KL, Berger PA, Hollister LE: Choline for tardive dyskinesia. *N Engl J Med* 293:152, 1975.

94. Miller E: Deanol in the treatment of levodopa-induced dyskinesias. *Neurology* 24:116–119, 1974.

95. Casey DE, Denney D: Dimethylaminoethanol in tardive dyskinesia. *N Engl J Med* 291:797, 1974.

96. Hanin I, Kopp U, Zahniser NR, et al: Acetylcholine and choline in human plasma and red blood cells: A gas chromatograph mass spectrometric evaluation, in Jenden DJ (ed): *Cholinergic Mechanisms and Psychopharmacology. Adv Behav Biol,* vol 24. New York, Plenum, 1977, pp 181–195.

97. Casey DE: Deanol in the management of involuntary movement disorders: A review. *Dis Nerv Syst* 38 (section 2):7–15, 1977.

98. Growdon JH, Hirsch MJ, Wurtman RJ, et al: Oral choline administration to patients with tardive dyskinesia. *N Engl J Med* 297:524–527, 1977.

99. Tamminga C, Smith RC, Erickson SE, et al: Cholinergic influences in tardive dyskinesia. *Am J Psychiatry* 134:769–774, 1977.

100. Growdon JH, Gelenberg AJ, Doller J, et al: Lecithin can suppress tardive dyskinesia. *N Engl J Med* 298:1029–1030, 1978.

101. Gelenberg AJ, Doller-Wojcik JC, Growdon JH: Choline and lecithin in the treatment of tardive dyskinesia: Preliminary results from a pilot study. *Am J Psychiatry* 136:772–776, 1979.

102. Jackson IV, Davis JG, Cohen RK, et al: Lecithin administration in tardive dyskinesia: Clinical and biomedical correlates. *Biol Psychiatry* 16:85–90, 1981.

103. Pradhan SN, Bose S: Interactions among central neurotransmitters, in Lipton MA, DiMascio A, Killam KF (eds): *Psychopharmacology: A Generation of Progress.* New York, Raven Press, 1978, pp 271–282.

104. Tamminga CA, Crayton JW, Chase TN: Improvement in tardive dyskinesia after muscimol therapy. *Arch Gen Psychiatry* 36:595–598, 1979.

105. Tamminga CA, Crayton JW, Chase TN: Muscimol: GABA agonist therapy in schizophrenia. *Am J Psychiatry* 135:746–747, 1978.

106. Casey DE, Gerlach J, Magelund G, et al: Gamma-acetylenic GABA in tardive dyskinesia. *Arch Gen Psychiatry* 37:1376–1379, 1980.

107. Linnoila M, Viukari M, Hietala O: Effect of sodium valproate on tardive dyskinesia. *Br J Psychiatry* 129:114–119, 1976.

108. Chien CP, Jung K, Ross-Townsend A: Efficacies of agents related to GABA, dopamine, and acetylcholine in the treatment of tardive dyskinesia. *Psychopharmacol Bull* 14:20–22, 1978.

109. Gibson AC: Sodium valproate and tardive dyskinesia. *Br J Psychiatry* 133:82, 1978.

110. Casey DE, Hammerstad JP: Sodium valproate in tardive dyskinesia. *J Clin Psychiatry* 40:483–485, 1979.

111. Nair NPV, Lal S, Schwartz G, et al: Effect of sodium valproate and baclofen in tardive dyskinesia: Clinical and neuroendocrine studies, in Cattabeni F, Racagni G, Spano PF, et al (eds): *Long-Term Effects of Neuroleptics. Adv Biochem Psychopharmacol,* vol 24. New York, Raven Press, 1980, pp 437–441.

112. Korsgaard S: Baclofen (Lioresal) in the treatment of neuroleptic-induced tardive dyskinesia. *Acta Psychiatr Scand* 54:17–24, 1976.

113. Gerlach J, Rye T, Kristjansen P: Effect of baclofen on tardive dyskinesia. *Psychopharmacol* 56:145–151, 1978.

114. Jus K, Jus A, Gautier J, et al: Studies on the action of certain pharmacological agents on tardive dyskinesia and on the rabbit syndrome. *Int J Clin Pharmacol* 9:138–145, 1974.

115. Singh MM: Diazepam in the treatment of tardive dyskinesia. *Int Pharmacopsychiatry* 11:232–234, 1976.

116. Singh MM, Nasrallah HA, Lal H, et al: Treatment of tardive dyskinesia with diazepam: Indirect evidence for the involvement of limbic, possibly GABAergic mechanisms. *Brain Res Bull* (suppl 2)5:673–680, 1980.

117. Rosenbaum AH, de la Fuente JR: Benzodiazepines and tardive dyskinesia. *Lancet* 2:900, 1979.

118. Sedman G: Clonazepam in treatment of tardive oral dyskinesia. *Br Med J* 2:583, 1976.

119. Bobruff A, Gardos G, Tarsy D, et al: Clonazepam and phenobarbital in tardive dyskinesia. *Am J Psychiatry* 138:189–193, 1981.

120. Bjørndal N, Casey DE, Gerlach J: Enkephalin, morphine, and naloxone in tardive dyskinesia. *Psychopharmacol* 69:133–136, 1980.

121. Casey DE, Korsgaard S, Gerlach J, et al: Effect of des-tyrosine-γ-endorphin in tardive dyskinesia. *Arch Gen Psychiatry* 38:158–160, 1981.

122. Tamminga CA, Tighe PJ, Chase TN, et al: Des-tyrosine-γ-endorphin administration in chronic schizophrenics. *Arch Gen Psychiatry* 38:167–168, 1981.

123. Gerlach J, Thorsen K, Munkvad I: Effect of lithium on neuroleptic-induced tardive dyskinesia compared with placebo in a double-blind crossover trial. *Pharmakopsychiatr Neuropsychopharmacol* 8:51–56, 1975.

124. Reda YF, Escobar JI, Scanlon JM: Lithium carbonate in the treatment of tardive dyskinesia. *Am J Psychiatry* 132:560–562, 1975.

125. Gardos G, Cole JO, Sniffen C: An evaluation of papaverine in tardive dyskinesia. *J Clin Pharmacol* 16:304–310, 1976.

126. Villeneuve A, Langlier P, Bedard P: Estrogens, dopamine and dyskinesias. *Can Psych Assoc J* 23:68–70, 1978.

127. Bedard PJ, Langelier P, Dankova J, et al: Estrogens, progesterone, and the extrapyramidal system, in Poirier LJ, Sourkes TL, Bedard PJ (eds): *Advances in Neurology,* vol 24. New York, Raven Press, 1979, pp 411–422.

128. Gomez E: Clinical observations in the treatment of tardive dyskinesia with dihydrogenated ergot alkaloids (Hydergine), preliminary findings. *Psychiatr J Univ Ottawa* 2:67–71, 1977.

129. Goldman D: Treatment of phenothiazine-induced dyskinesia. *Psychopharmacol* 47:271–272, 1976.

130. Prange AJ, Wilson IC, Morris CE, et al: Preliminary experience with tryptophan and lithium in the treatment of tardive dyskinesia. *Psychopharmacol Bull* 9:36, 1973.

131. Vale S, Espejel MA: Amantadine for dyskinesia tarda. *N Engl J Med* 284:1091, 1971.

132. Crane GE: More about the use of amantadine in tardive dyskinesia. *N Engl J Med* 285:1150, 1971.

133. Janowsky DS, El-Yousef MK, Davis JM, et al: Effects of amantadine on tardive dyskinesia and pseudoparkinsonism. *N Engl J Med* 286:785, 1972.

134. Fann WE, Davis JM, Wilson IC: Methylphenidate in tardive dyskinesia. *Am J Psychiatry* 130:922–924, 1973.

135. DeVeaugh-Geiss J, Manion L: High-dose pyridoxine in tardive dyskinesia. *J Clin Psychiatry* 39:573–575, 1978.

136. Crane GE, Turek IS, Kurland AA: Failure of pyridoxine to reduce drug-induced dyskinesias. *J Neurol Neurosurg Psychiatry* 33:511–512, 1970.

137. Freedman R, Bell J, Kirch D: Clonidine therapy for coexisting psychosis and tardive dyskinesia. *Am J Psychiatry* 137:629–630, 1980.

138. Bacher NM, Lewis HA: Low-dose propranolol in tardive dyskinesia. *Am J Psychiatry* 137:495–497, 1980.

9 Neuroleptic-Induced Supersensitivity Psychosis

Guy Chouinard

During our standardized long-term neuroleptic treatment of 300 schizophrenic patients over the last eight years, we have noticed that a significant proportion of our patients become quite paranoid one or two days before their routine injection of depot neuroleptics. These are patients who are otherwise well maintained on their medications, are considered to be in remission, and often are still employed at the same job they had before they became ill. This observation, plus the results from some of our controlled drug trials of neuroleptic withdrawal in schizophrenic patients, led us to suggest the possibility of a drug-induced psychosis, and eventually to formulate the hypothesis of supersensitivity psychosis.[1]

Supersensitivity psychosis, like tardive dyskinesia, is a supersensitivity syndrome induced by long-term use of neuroleptic drugs. It consists of positive symptoms of schizophrenia, eg, suspiciousness, delusions, thought disorders or hallucinations.[2] Like tardive dyskinesia, supersensitivity psychosis has pharmacologic characteristics that are associated with a postsynaptic dopamine receptor supersensitivity.[3]

1. The symptoms appear when neuroleptics are discontinued, when dosage is reduced, or in the case of depot neuroleptics, at the end of the injection interval.
2. The syndrome appears only after a history of at least a few weeks of treatment with neuroleptics and is best seen after several months of neuroleptic treatment.
3. Concomitant signs of dopamine supersensitivity such as tardive dyskinesia are often present. However, some patients, especially those with a poor prognosis in long-term wards of mental hospitals, may develop severe tardive dyskinesia upon withdrawal of neuroleptics and not display signs of supersensitivity psychosis, suggesting that there may no longer be sufficient dopamine available to produce positive symptoms in those areas of brain involved with the schizophrenic pyschosis.
4. The syndrome is associated with a sudden fall in prolactin levels when neuroleptics are discontinued, suggesting that the appearance of the supersensitivity psychosis is associated with the decrease in the dopamine-blocking effect of the neuroleptics.
5. The syndrome is associated with central nervous system (CNS) tolerance to antipsychotic effects; ie, a gradual increase in neuroleptic dosage is necessary to maintain a therapeutic effect. The CNS drug tolerance is best seen in patients receiving high doses of neuroleptics and those who are considered drug responders.
6. As with tardive dyskinesia, the most efficacious treatment is the causative agent itself, the neuroleptic. In most cases, the neuroleptic will produce rapid improvement.

There are some difficulties associated with the diagnosis of supersensitivity psychosis. First, the symptoms are nearly the same as the original illness; the distinction being that only positive symptoms of schizophrenia are exhibited and that they disappear immediately after receiving the medication. Also, relapse occurs more rapidly than would be expected after cessation of neuroleptic therapy. Second, the clinical symptoms are covered up by the medication itself. Patients on IM long-acting medication only display the symptoms at the end of the injection interval; for those patients on oral neuroleptics, one must rely on the patient's account of the events following a missed dose. Third, medications such as chlorpromazine have an effect on the adrenergic, histamine, and serotoninergic systems, which make it difficult to distinguish side effects from supersensitivity psychosis when the medication is discontinued or decreased. Patients treated with low potency neuroleptics such as chlor-promazine or thioridazine will complain of insomnia, nausea and of restlessness when they missed or stopped their medication. This should not be confused with supersensitivity psychosis since these effects are related more to the cholinergic rebound effect. Fourth, the syndrome is more easily recognized in good prognosis patients. Fifth, supersensitivity psychosis will be best seen in patients under stress of normal life. Recent animal studies indicate that stress may increase supersensitivity.[4]

The diagnostic criteria of the syndrome are the following:

1. It consists only of positive symptoms of schizophrenia: suspiciousness, delusions, thought disorders or hallucinations. Acute catatonic symptoms may be seen, but are rare.
2. The positive symptoms of the original illness must be in complete remission at one time in order to speak of an appearance.
3. It is only when dosage is reduced, medication stopped or at the end of the injection period for those only on injectable neuroleptics that the symptoms will appear.
4. Their appearance is sudden.
5. Their response to neuroleptics is dramatic; within 24 hours the symptoms have completely disappeared.
6. Contrary to tardive dyskinesia, which is not readily reversible, supersensitivity psychosis is more readily reversible through desensitization by gradual decrease of the neuroleptics. The desensitization needs to be done gradually, not more than 5% of the dose per two to three weeks. Desensitization by small dose reduction supports the supersensitivity origin of the disorder. The greater reversibility of the syndrome is not surprising in view of recent animal studies showing high dopamine turnover in cell bodies of mesolimbic regions.[5]

We hypothesize that supersensitivity psychosis is caused by supersensitivity of the dopaminergic receptor in the mesolimbic regions, or other dopaminergic regions that would be related to psychotic symptoms. Such a supersensitivity has been shown to develop in animals upon administration of neuroleptics,[6] and there have been reports of an increase of dopamine-binding sites in the mesolimbic region of the brains of schizophrenic patients.[7]

Although this is still theoretical at this stage, we try to distinguish between positive and negative symptoms of schizophrenia, arguing that an increase in dopamine-binding sites in the mesolimbic, which is responsible for supersensitivity psychosis, is related to positive symptoms, as is seen, for example, in amphetamine psychosis.[1] Conversely, a decrease in dopaminergic function in this region, either by the blocking action of neuroleptics or dopamine-depleting drugs, is related to the negative symptoms. In this model, negative symptoms subside through supersensitivity for those patients who show improvement. In contrast, those patients whose negative symptoms do not improve significantly may develop supersensitivity in other regions of the brain such as in the neostriatum, and are more likely to develop tardive dyskinesia and, probably because of their poor therapeutic response, these patients are likely to receive higher doses of neuroleptic drugs. This lack of therapeutic response also could be explained through the absence of supersensitivity and, therefore, explain the absence of supersensitivity psychosis. This hypothesis further argues that supersensitivity in the neostriatum is responsible for tardive dyskinesia, while a decrease in dopaminergic function in that area induces parkinsonism.

In order to accept this idea of a supersensitivity psychosis it is necessary to show that there is CNS drug tolerance to the therapeutic effect of the neuroleptic medications.[8] Tolerance to the therapeutic effect of neuroleptics is a complicated issue. There are some prerequisites for tolerance to develop. First, it should be stated that it is not a metabolic tolerance but a tolerance related to supersensitivity induced by neuroleptics. One condition for supersensitivity is that patients receive sufficiently high doses of neuroleptic so that when it is decreased or discontinued, the syndrome is more evident. Second, patients must have recovered from their original illness and be in remission. Patients who are chronically hallucinating and in long-term wards of mental hospitals will display the syndrome less. That patients with poor prognoses are less likely to produce the syndrome may be because there is little dopamine reaching receptor sites or there is a defective receptor response. The matter is more complicated when we consider that the tolerance or supersensitivity induced by neuroleptics in the mesolimbic regions could also have a therapeutic effect on the negative symptoms. Thus, it is only those symptoms that respond quickly to neuroleptics through their dopamine-blocking effect that are going to reappear. Finally, stress is important to uncover supersensitivity. Supersensitivity psychosis will be most likely to be seen in those patients who are outside the hospital and under normal stressful situations of life.

In a double-blind controlled study of seven months' duration, we compared fluphenazine enanthate given every two weeks with fluphenazine decanoate given every four weeks in the maintenance treatment of 48 schizophrenic outpatients.[9] Before entering the trial, patients had received fluphenazine enanthate routinely for periods of 1 to 108 months (median: 15). All patients underwent a further one-month period of stabilization with enanthate: the bimonthly dosages ranging from 2.5 to 125 mg (geometric mean: 25 mg). Twenty-four patients were assigned to each treatment at random. During the study, the dosages of either drug were adjusted according to therapeutic response. Twelve patients (50%) treated with decanoate and nine (37.5%) treated with enanthate required gradual increases in dosage. By week 28, there had been significant (p < .01) increases in the geometric mean doses of decanoate (range: 2.5 to 250 mg; mean: 32.1 mg) and enanthate (range: 2.5 to 325 mg; mean: 40.2 mg). Thus, substantial increases in dosage were required to maintain the mean therapeutic effect at the same level. In animal studies, prolonged exposure to neuroleptics leads to increased dosage requirements to block the behavioral effects of apomorphine.[10,11]

A number of clinical considerations followed from this work: 1) The existence of supersensitivity psychosis may explain Hogarty's finding that two thirds of patients thought to be most suitable for drug withdrawal after two years of drug therapy relapsed following drug discontinuation, causing the authors to state "the need for maintenance chemotherapy may be indefinite."[12] 2) Since those who are the most responsive to neuroleptics are also those who are more likely to develop supersensitivity psychosis, good prognosis schizophrenic patients should be treated with neuroleptics with a less potent therapeutic effect on the acute symptoms such as pimozide,[13] penfluridol,[14] or fluspirilene.[15] 3) For the outpatient treatment of schizophrenic patients, the clinician must avoid the vicious circle of increasing the medication for those patients on injectable neuroleptics who, when seen at the end of the injection period, are paranoid at the time of interview. Also, medication should not be increased in female patients who, during menstruation, become paranoid or hallucinate, since these symptoms may be part of the supersensitivity psychosis, and increasing the dose will lead to increased supersensitivity.

In a preliminary study of the incidence of supersensitivity psychosis, we estimate the syndrome to be present in 30% of chronically treated schizophrenic patients; those who tend to develop the syndrome appear more frequently in the good prognosis group, as opposed to those who tend to develop tardive dyskinesia, although there is an overlap. A recent report on withdrawal of neuroleptics showed that it is in the first three weeks of neuroleptic withdrawal that there is a difference in the relapse rate between those patients who are continued on neuroleptics and those who are discontinued.[16] Those with an early relapse are those who are most likely to have supersensitivity psychosis. In the same study, the relationship between relapse rate and tardive dyskinesia was studied. It was found that although the relationship between the two syndromes appeared to be in the "expected direction," the correlation was not statistically significant. In our original study,[3] we found the two syndromes to be correlated; our latest work on the subject shows that they are not necessarily associated for a given patient. Supersensitivity psychosis tends to be associated with good prognosis patients and tardive dyskinesia was more severe in poor prognosis patients.

Another recent study on neuroleptic withdrawal with fluphenazine decanoate reports that 80% of their 47 patients relapsed on withdrawal of neuroleptics (half during withdrawal itself and half after withdrawal).[17] In the same study, the authors report a significant difference in symptomatology between the patients who relapsed during withdrawal and those who relapsed after withdrawal of the neuroleptic: patients relapsing during withdrawal exhibited significantly more symptoms, which are different from those of their original illness, than those relapsing after withdrawal.

In conclusion, 30% to 40% of patients showed rapid relapse upon withdrawal of neuroleptics, a type of relapse compatible with supersensitivity psychosis. Recognition of the syndrome is important in order to avoid escalating the dosage. Supersensitivity psychosis appears to differ from tardive dyskinesia in terms of patients more likely to present the disorder. Supersensitivity psychosis also appears more readily reversible than tardive dyskinesia.

ACKNOWLEDGMENT

The author wishes to thank Elaine Lewis, MA for her assistance with the editing of the manuscript.

REFERENCES

1. Chouinard G, Jones BD: Schizophrenia as dopamine-deficiency disease. *Lancet* 2:99–100, 1978.

2. Chouinard G, Jones BD: Neuroleptic-induced supersensitivity psychosis: Clinical and pharmacologic characteristics. *Am J Psychiatry* 137:16–21, 1980.

3. Chouinard G, Jones BD, Annable L: Neuroleptic-induced supersensitivity psychosis. *Am J Psychiatry* 135:1409–1410, 1978.

4. Antelman SM, Eichler AJ, Black CA, et al: Interchangeability of stress and amphetamine in sensitization. *Science* 207:329–331, 1980.

5. Agnati LF, Fuxe K, Anderson K, et al: The mesolimbic dopamine system: Evidence for a high amine turnover and for a heterogeneity of the dopamine neuron population. *Neurosci Lett* 18:45–51, 1980.

6. Seeger TF, Gardner IL: Enhancement of self-stimulation behavior in rats and monkeys after chronic neuroleptic treatment: Evidence for mesolimbic supersensitivity. *Brain Res* 175:49–57, 1979.

7. Owen F, Cross AJ, Crow TJ, et al: Increased dopamine receptor sensitivity in schizophrenia. *Lancet* 2:223–226, 1979.

8. Chouinard G, Jones BD, Annable L: Neuroleptic-induced supersensitivity psychosis, in Usdin E, Eckert H, Forrest IS (eds): *Phenothiazines and Structurally Related Drugs: Basic and Clinical Studies, Developments in Neuroscience,* vol 7. New York, Elsevier, 1980.

9. Chouinard G, Annable L, Ross-Chouinard A: Comparison of fluphenazine esters in the treatment of schizophrenic outpatients: Extrapyramidal symptoms and therapeutic effect. *Am J Psychiatry* (in press).

10. Asper H, Baggiolini M, Burki HR, et al: Tolerance phenomena with neuroleptics: Catalepsy, apomorphine stereotypes and striatal dopamine metabolism in the rat after single and repeated administration of loxapine and haloperidol. *Eur J Pharmacol* 22:287–294, 1973.

11. Møller Nielson I, Fajalland B, Pedersen V, et al: Pharmacology of neuroleptics upon repeated administration. *Psychopharmacologia (Berl)* 34:95–104, 1974.

12. Hogarty GE, Ulrich RF, Mussare F, et al: Drug discontinuation among longterm successfully maintained schizophrenic outpatients. *Dis Nerv Syst* 37:494–500, 1976.

13. Chouinard G, Annable L: Pimozide in the treatment of acute schizophrenia. *The 132nd Annual Meeting of the American Psychiatric Association Abstracts.* Chicago, 1979, pp 247–248.

14. Chouinard G, Annable L: Penfluridol in the treatment of newly admitted schizophrenic patients in a brief therapy unit. *Am J Psychiatry* 133:820–823, 1976.

15. Chouinard G, Annable L, Denis JF: Fluspirilene in the treatment of acute schizophrenia. *Scientific Proceedings from 30th Annual Meeting of the Canadian Psychiatric Association.* Toronto, October 1–3, 1980.

16. Levine J, Schooler NR, Severe, J, et al: Discontinuation of oral and depot fluphenazine in schizophrenic patients after one year of continuous medication: A controlled study. *Adv Biochem Psychopharmacol* 24:483–493, 1980.

17. Capstick N: Long-term fluphenazine decanoate maintenance dosage requirements of chronic schizophrenic patients. *Acta Psychiatr Scand* 61:256–262, 1980.

10 Gilles de la Tourette's Syndrome

Eric D. Caine

In the last 15 years, psychiatric researchers in the United States have questioned the accuracy of clinical diagnoses. Investigators have frequently reclassified patients from one diagnostic cluster to another. Mindful of this state of flux, I decided to study those neuropsychiatric disorders that would lend themselves to more reliable discrimination. In addition to such syndromes as Huntington's disease (with its movement disorder, dementia, and prominent psychopathology) and behavior disorders due to focal brain lesions, Gilles de la Tourette's syndrome appeared to provide a useful neuropsychiatric *model* for more common functional disorders. The response of many patients to haloperidol, the precise diagnostic criteria, and the combination of movement and behavioral symptoms in one syndrome, presented what appeared to be an ideal setting for clinical and pharmacological research.

This chapter will review a series of clinical investigations conducted in collaboration with colleagues from the National Institute of Mental Health. They indicate this disorder may result from a variety of neurochemical abnormalities, suggesting that more than one patho-physiological mechanism may lead to the expression of the distinctive symptom cluster we call Gilles de la Tourette's syndrome.

At the time we began our efforts, Drs Arthur and Elaine Shapiro and their co-workers had already provided the outlines of the prominent features of Tourette's syndrome (TS). Other investigators had also described the disorder, although in smaller numbers. From the work of our predecessors, we attempted to select those core clinical criteria that would adequately identify potential research subjects. These included: 1) the presence of multiple motor and vocal tics; 2) onset before age 14 years; 3) a waxing and waning course; and 4) the gradual disappearance of old symptoms with a replacement by new ones. Signs and symptoms that were found in other abnormal involuntary movement disorders (eg, exacerbation of symptoms by stress or the ability to suppress movements voluntarily for brief periods) were not regarded as core features, although they were uniformly present in the patients that we ultimately studied. Motor tics were defined as sudden, rapid, repetitive, involuntary movements of a stereotyped nature. Vocal tics involved motor movements, which led to the emanation of involuntary sounds, frequently including grunts, clicks, throat-clearing, inhalations, exhalations (snorts), shouts, squeals, words, obscenities, stereotyped phrases, and jargon.

Among the questions we chose to address were the following: Is TS a genetic disorder? What are some of the factors that contribute to the heterogeneity of patient response to haloperidol? What are the consequences that arise when patients take this potent neuroleptic for extended periods? Is there a documentable neurophysiological abnormality that corresponds to the complaint by many Tourette patients that they have difficulty sleeping? Are other medications available for treating Tourette's syndrome that have less acute toxicity or long-term risk than haloperidol?

CLINICAL INVESTIGATIONS

Several researchers have suggested that Tourette's syndrome is a genetically mediated disorder,[1,2] although others have questioned this premise.[3] As part of our comprehensive study, we systematically collected the family histories of the first 50 patients identified in the NIH clinic as having TS.[4] Data were gathered concerning 2,139 patients and relatives. The patients' areas of residence and religious backgrounds were not substantially different from those of all patients referred to NIH from 1975 to 1977. The entire range of the socioeconomic spectrum was represented in the population, as well. There was no preponderance of individuals with a Jewish, eastern European background, as had been found in earlier studies from New York City, where the individuals sampled were drawn from a specific geographic area that had an unusually high number of individuals with that heritage. In addition to assessing family history, we ascertained the presence of a number of *associated* behaviors in the Tourette patients, including obsessive-compulsive behavior as defined by DSM-III, learning disabilities, sleep difficulties, self-mutilating or self-destructive behavior, inappropriate sexual activity, and impulsive/antisocial behaviors. The latter two clusters were not sought initially, but the spontaneous observation or reporting of these dysfunctions suggested that a more careful survey was in order.

We found that 16 families contained a member other than the proband who had TS. Another 16 families had at least one individual who had motor tics; in these families the proband was the only member with the full syndrome. A third group of 18 families had no history of any individual other than the proband having TS, motor tics, or vocal tics. There was no significant difference between family groups in the frequency of neurological illnesses, alcoholism, and ethnic or geographic origin. There was a tendency for both speech problems and emotional problems to occur more commonly in association with tics or TS in the family tree ($p < 0.05$ for both disorders), although the amount of variance explained by these relationships was quite small and thus difficult to interpret. It was of note that a number of family members described historically the spontaneous remission of tics or Tourette's syndrome. This finding suggested that Tourette's syndrome or the tic disorder, which commonly appears in the family members of Tourette patients, is not uniformly life-long, although it is persistent in many individuals.

The characteristics of the 50 patients are summarized in Table 10-1. The age of onset ranged from 2 to 13 years, with a mean of 7.0 years. This is in accord with previous findings.[5] Coprolalia was present in 29 of the 50 (58%), which was also similar to samples collected by Shapiro and colleagues. Of note was a high occurrence of obsessive-compulsive behaviors, self-destructive behaviors, and frequent but less common, inappropriate sexual activity and antisocial behavior. Learning disabilities were common, as were sleep disturbances.

These associated behaviors are defined rigidly in order to avoid confusion and "impressionistic" classification.[4] Our results suggest that Tourette's syndrome is characterized by a number of behavioral difficulties that are not often included as core diagnostic symptoms. These abnormalities are not uncommon in other neuropsychiatric disorders, however, nor are they sufficient to establish the presence of Tourette's

Table 10-1
Characteristics of 50 Patients with Tourette's Syndrome*

Feature	No. of Patients
Tourette-related characteristic	
Coprolalia	29
Sleep disturbance	22
Learning disability	20
Obsessive-compulsive behavior	34
Self-destructive behavior	24
Inappropriate sexual activity	16
Antisocial behavior	13
Haloperidol response (N = 46)	
Positive	31
Variable	11
Negative	4
Reported side effects	25
No side effects	21

*Reprinted by permission of *Ann Neurol* 7:41–49, 1980.

syndrome. They point to the possibility that the neurochemical pathophysiology which underlies TS may also account for other, more common functional disturbances. Alternatively, behaviors such as obsessions, compulsions, or learning disabilities may be "final common pathways" for a variety of distinct pathophysiological processes.

Table 10-2 illustrates the relationship between therapeutic response to haloperidol and family history. A positive family history for TS, or a family history of tics, is associated strongly with a positive response to haloperidol. Some patients demonstrate a *variable* response to this medication. They benefit from pharmacotherapy when their symptoms are on the wane, but many show little benefit or markedly increased side effects when the medication is raised in response to periodic symptom exacerbation. Side effects are least common among those individuals with a positive family history for TS and most apparent in those individuals who have no affected relatives.

The findings from this painstaking family history survey indicate that some patients have a genetically transmitted disorder. The data do not easily conform to a simplified model of genetic transmission. Taken together with the patients' responses to haloperidol (a clinical "neuropharmacological provocation test"), we get a picture of a heterogeneous disorder, with "haloperidol-responsive" and "haloperidol-nonresponsive" neurochemical abnormalities.

During the family history survey, it became apparent that a number of individuals complained of disordered sleep. Six of these patients (five

Table 10-2
Haloperidol Response in 46 Patients with Tourette's Syndrome*

Response	Patients with Family History of: Tourette's Syndrome (N = 15)	Tics (N = 16)	Patients with Negative Family History (N = 15)	X²	% Variance[a]
Therapeutic response					
Positive	14	11	6	X² = 10.57, p<0.01	23
Variable	0	4	7	...	...
Negative	1	1	2	...	...
Side effects at all doses					
Reported	4	9	12	X² = 8.63, p<0.02	19
Not reported	11	7	3	...	...
Side effects at 5 mg or less	(N=9)	(N=7)	(N=11)		
Reported	3	4	11	X² = 10.28, p<0.01	38
Not reported	6	3	0		

[a]Percent of variance accounted for by X² at this level of significance.
*Reprinted by permission of *Ann Neurol* 7:41–49, 1980.

unequivocal responders to haloperidol and one variable responder) were examined in the sleep laboratory of the National Institute of Mental Health.[6] Sleep EEG data indicated that these individuals, who had been maintained without medication for at least three weeks, had 30% less delta sleep (stages 3 and 4 combined) than a group of nine normal volunteers matched for age and sex ratio ($p < 0.05$). When the patients were given haloperidol, there was a marked increase in delta sleep time and percentage ($p < 0.01$), to an extent that the sleep times of the patients were indistinguishable from those of the volunteers.

This definable alteration of sleep, and its improvement following haloperidol therapy, provides a documentable neurophysiological parallel to the motor and behavior abnormalities discussed previously. We appear to be dealing with one or more neurochemical disorders manifest at multiple levels of the central nervous system, affecting at once basic biological rhythms, motor control, and complex behaviors. With this great variety of symptoms, we may be observing the results of an ascending neurochemical modulating system gone awry.

COMPLICATIONS OF HALOPERIDOL THERAPY

Pharmacotherapy with haloperidol may have significant complications in some TS patients. In 1978, we described a 15-year-old with the onset of tardive dyskinesia following the discontinuation of a daily medication regimen that included: haloperidol, 50 mg; amitriptyline, 150 mg; and trihexyphenidyl, 2 mg.[7] He demonstrated typical oral-facial dyskinesia, in addition to dyskinetic movements of the trunk and marked choreoathetosis of the upper and lower extremities. His truncal dyskinesia was severe enough to cause great difficulty with tandem stance or gait. By the fourth week following drug discontinuation, his oral, facial, and lower extremity movements had diminished, but his marked choreoathetosis of the upper extremities and trunk remained constant.

Beginning with the fourth week following drug discontinuation, the patient began to show signs of disordered thought form and content; his symptoms evolved to the point that he demonstrated a marked loss of ability to concentrate, highly personalized and bizarre delusions (including delusions of omnipotence and grandeur), and he described experiences of déjà vu, déjà écouté, and depersonalization. He manifested frequent derailment. Ultimately, the patient required haloperidol elixir, 60 mg daily, before he experienced a gradual remission of symptoms. It was possible that this young man demonstrated a tardive psychosis, in addition to his tardive dyskinesia (see Chapter 9). Since evaluating this individual, my colleagues and I have recommended that patients be monitored for early signs of abnormal involuntary movements at least once every three to four months. We have encountered three other individuals with tardive dyskinesia; in two, symptoms have remitted following drug discontinuation.[8]

Haloperidol may also lead to a drug-induced dysphoria.[9] This appears to be distinctive from the *akinetic* depressions that have been described recently in schizophrenia.[10] Those are thought to represent mild extrapyramidal reactions, with lack of spontaneity, masked facies and decreased arm swing. The patients we observed had none of these signs, nor any previous history of major affective disturbance. Each experienced the sudden onset of marked dysphoria following the increase of haloperidol past an apparent dosage *threshold*. One described it as follows: "It was as if a shade suddenly came down." In another individual who was participating in a double-blind experimental protocol, it was possible to establish with confidence that his changes were not related to a specific knowledge about the medication he was taking. Throughout the procedure, the number of tablets he received was unchanged. His dose was raised and lowered unbeknownst to him and the clinical rater; each time it was increased above 4 mg per day, he became inappropriately sad and tearful. He did not experience drowsiness, obvious cognitive impairment, akathisia, akinesia, or other extrapyramidal side effects. His mood improved markedly whenever the dose was decreased to 4 mg or less. From our clinical experience, it was apparent that as many as 10% of Tourette patients taking haloperidol may have encountered this disturbing dysphoria.

Haloperidol also causes measurable neuroendocrine changes, although the clinical significance of these is unknown.[11] An adolescent who had a delayed onset of puberty was investigated with all night sleep and endocrine studies, as we had concerns about the effect of haloperidol on his eventual growth and development. Prolactin, growth hormone, and luteinizing hormone were measured. Blood samples were collected every 20 minutes throughout each night of sleep through an intravenous catheter that had been connected to a ten-foot extension tubing. The patient was studied before treatment, on the tenth day of treatment when his dose was 5 mg po qhs (10 PM), and again on the 81st day of therapy, when the dose had been lowered to 2 mg po qhs. As seen in Table 10-3, there was no significant effect on growth hormone during either study night. However, prolactin was significantly increased on both occasions while luteinizing hormone was suppressed. The patient showed gradual progress in his pubertal changes, with an increase in testicular size and growth of axillary and pubic hair. In the year following the endocrine study, he demonstrated further growth of axillary, pubic, and facial hair, and phallic changes consistent with puberty. Although this young man appeared to experience no growth suppression from haloperidol, there were consistent, measurable changes in both prolactin and luteinizing hormone. The episodic pattern of their release continued despite the drug treatment. It was not possible to establish in this single case study whether quantitative alterations in the amount of hormone secreted led to clinically meaningful consequences. A single case study can raise our level of concern, but it cannot adequately assess or predict the kind of infrequent side effects that might only be present in an occasional individual.

Table 10-3
Mean Plasma Levels ($\pm$ SEM) of Prolactin (PRL),
Luteinizing Hormone (LH), and Growth Hormone (GH):
Pretreatment, Day 10, Day 81*

	Pretreatment	Day 10 $(p)^a$	Day 81 (p)
PRL (ng/ml)	16.0 ± 1.9	44.3 ± 2.2 (< .001)	30.2 ± 2.0 (< .001)
LH (mIU/ml)	9.4 ± 0.5	6.4 ± 0.6 (< .001)	8.0 ± 0.4 (< .05)
GH (ng/ml)	3.0 ± 0.8	2.8 ± 0.7 (NS)	2.5 ± 0.6 (NS)

[a]Two-tailed t-test for group means comparing mean hormone response to treatment *vs* pretreatment level.
*Reprinted by permission *J Nerv Ment Dis* 167:504–507, © 1979, Baltimore, The Williams & Wilkins Co.

THERAPEUTIC TRIALS WITH TOURETTE PATIENTS

Despite a well-defined set of diagnostic criteria and target symptoms which are countable, there are many obstacles that confront the investigator who wishes to perform pharmacotherapeutic trials with TS patients.

1. The disorder, by definition, changes spontaneously over time (a waxing and waning course). One must separate sustained, drug-induced improvement from a spontaneous remission for an extended period.
2. There is marked variation in the severity of tics throughout a day; when observed in a controlled format, a patient may manifest wide fluctuations of symptom intensity that are "statistically significant" (E.D. Caine, MD et al, unpublished data, 1981).
3. TS may be a pathophysiologically heterogeneous disorder; more than one neurochemical abnormality may lead to its final expression.
4. Patients with TS are extremely responsive to environmental or situational influences. This may be seen in: a) a dramatic decrease in tic frequency when a patient visits the doctor; b) an increase in symptom intensity during times of excitement or distress; c) a temporary decrease of symptoms with an active placebo (one that has side effects but no therapeutic effect); and d) the transient but impressive improvement of TS symptoms which can, at times, be brought forth by accurate diagnosis, physician support and counseling, and an enthusiastic, hopeful espousal of pharmacotherapeutic agents (the "physician placebo effect").

With these confounds in mind, a series of pharmacotherapeutic trials were undertaken in a highly controlled inpatient setting. Informed consent was obtained from all patients and from the parents of individuals under 18 years of age. Patients were assessed with a twice-weekly global rating and with twice-weekly tic counts (at the same time each day), during which a blind rater observed the patient engaged in conversation with another individual for a five-minute period. These patients were oriented to the study format during a baseline period to lessen their anxiety. The significance of changes in each of the Tourette patients' tic counts was evaluated with Wilcoxon's two-sample rank sum test.

Using this format, my colleagues and I assessed the efficacy of clozapine, chlorimipramine, desipramine, and lecithin for treating patients with Tourette's syndrome. Clozapine was selected as a potentially beneficial compound because it was the first non-neuroleptic antipsychotic agent; it reduced thought disorder without creating significant extrapyramidal symptoms. No patients using clozapine for extended periods of time have been described as having tardive dyskinesia. Seven TS patients participated in the protocol.[12] Unfortunately, there were no statistically significant improvements in either tic counts or clinical global ratings.

Chlorimipramine, a tricyclic antidepressant, blocks serotonin reuptake at the presynaptic neuron in a relatively specific manner in vitro.[13] It has been shown in man to increase the principal metabolite of serotonin (5-hydroxyindoleacetic acid) in cerebral spinal fluid.[14] Desipramine, a compound with a constellation of side effects similar to that of chlorimipramine, is a tricyclic antidepressant that blocks primarily the reuptake of norepinephrine while having little effect on serotonin.[13,15] It provides a useful contrast agent to chlorimipramine, with comparable side effects but distinct neurochemical action.

Yaryura-Tobias and Neziroglu[16] had suggested that chlorimipramine was a particularly efficacious agent in the treatment of Tourette symptoms. We studied this with a double-blind protocol, where six patients participated in a three-way trial; each received chlorimipramine, desipramine, and placebo.[17] The maximum daily dose of the two active drugs was 150 mg; medication was dispensed in 50 mg tablets. Each study phase lasted four weeks with a minimum of three days separating the phases.

There were no statistically significant or clinically significant improvements in patients' tic frequency throughout the study (Table 10-4). The clinical condition of one patient deteriorated rapidly while taking chlorimipramine, while the other five showed no substantial change. These results suggested that there may have been little serotoninergic contribution to the neurochemical pathophysiology of the TS symptoms in five of our subjects. The sixth, who showed a marked exacerbation of his symptoms, may have had an abnormality where serotonin was involved in the neurochemical mediation of the disorder. Desipramine had neither a therapeutic nor an exacerbating influence on the five patients who ultimately received it. This suggested a lack of norepinephrine-mediated abnormality in these individuals.

Lecithin was studied in light of recent interest in the cholinergic control of motor function[18] (see also Chapter 13). Six patients (different ones from the prior trials) participated in this double-blind, cross-over study. Each was given a maximum daily dose of 45 gm of lecithin (Lethicon, American Lecithin Co, 55% phosphatidyl choline), which

Table 10-4
Patient Characteristics: Response to Chlorimipramine (CLI) and Desipramine (DMI)*

Patient No., Sex, and Age (yr)	Clinical Features	CLI			DMI	
		Tic Count[a]	Response	Tic Count	Response	Tic Count
1. M, 16	Simple tics, vocal tics, coprolalia	55.0 (6.2)	Marked symptom exacerbation; symptoms abated when medication discontinued after 9 days	None	No symptom change; initial marked somnolence	50.1 (13.7)
2. M, 31	Simple and complex tics, vocal tics	14.7 (5.8)	No symptom change; initial complaints of "racing thoughts, nervous feelings"	17.7 (8.1)	...	...
3. M, 24	Simple and complex tics, vocal tics, coprolalia	88.8 (13.1)	No symptom change; persistent blurred vision, initial difficulty sleeping, initial GI distress	106.0 (21.6)	No symptom change; no side-effects	83.4 (14.9)

4. M, 16	Simple and complex tics, vocal tics, coprolalia	107.8 (19.6)	No symptom change; orthostatic hypotension during first 2 weeks	138.0 (37.9)	No symptom change; no side-effects	116.8 (63.2)
5. F, 13	Simple and complex tics, choreoathetoid movements, vocal tics, coprolalia	74.6 (13.1)	Mild increase in tics (not statistically significant); complaints of dry mouth	97.6 (14.2)	No symptom change; complaints of dry mouth	75.3 (17.7)
6. M, 15	Simple tics, vocal tics	13.0 (9.1)	No symptom change; complaints of mild to moderate shortness of breath after athletic exertion	15.2 (4.2)	No symptom change; persistent blurred vision, initial somnolence	19.5 (4.6)

[a]Tic count: mean tic count on either placebo, chlorimipramine, or desipramine phase (1 standard deviation).

*Reprinted by permission from *Ann Neurol* 5:305–306, 1979.

was administered for four weeks. They were also given a similar-appearing placebo. In addition to motor tic assessment, vocal tics were tape-recorded for evaluation. Each patient was assessed for five minutes per rating, with three minutes of conversation and two minutes of reading aloud. Vocal tics were counted by "blind" listeners from tape recordings of these sessions.

Lecithin induced a variety of individual responses, but there was no discernible benefit for the group as a whole (see Table 10-5). No important side effects were observed during the study. The minor improvements in two patients as well as deterioration of two others could be explained by heterogeneous neurochemical pathophysiologies, or the spontaneous waxing and waning of tics. These findings, using high doses of an acetylcholine precursor, suggested that cholinergic augmentation may prove beneficial for occasional individuals, but it appears to have no therapeutic effect for many TS patients.

Table 10-5
Cholinergic Treatment in Tourette's Syndrome*

Patient No.	Sex/ Age (yr)	Motor-Tic Counts†			Vocal-Tic Counts†		
		Placebo	*Lecithin*	*P Value*	*Placebo*	*Lecithin*	*P Value*
1	F/12	91.1	77.4	0.05	76.6	87.1	NS‡
2	F/20	60.5	56.3	NS‡	71.4	93.7	0.005
3	F/30	89.2	83.9	NS‡	13.5	12.2	NS‡
4	M/13	19.0	17.6	NS‡	55.7	36.8	0.001
5	M/13	85.0	Status tic§	—	96.9	33.5	0.02
6	M/69	111.8	Status tic§	—	4.6	12.8	0.001

*Reprinted by permission of *N Engl J Med* 302:1310, 1980.
†Tic counts expressed as mean number of tics in five minutes.
‡NS denotes not significant.
§Status tic refers to continuous tic activity too rapid to quantify.

Pharmacotherapy trials with small numbers of patients with a syndrome such as TS encounter another major difficulty. Investigations with relatively few subjects may fail to detect a therapeutic effect that occurs in a small percentage of affected individuals. It is also difficult to recognize outliers when the groups are as small as the ones we investigated. There is also the tendency to study the same individuals repeatedly when one is dealing with a relatively rare disorder. These deficiencies point to the need for large cooperative studies where investigators employ standardized protocols, with carefully constructed measures of motor and vocal tic frequency. Moreover, it will be necessary to carefully consider the responses of each patient, with an eye to detecting what might be termed "unique responders."

CONCLUSION

This chapter has attempted to present an overview of a variety of clinical studies devoted to unraveling the pathophysiology of TS and discovering drugs to treat it more effectively. The early assumption that this uncommon, distinctive syndrome represents a relatively homogeneous disorder must be questioned. Indeed, one may want to reverse that assumption at the present time, maintaining an operational stance that the symptoms we encounter are a "final common pathway" for a variety of neurochemical pathophysiologies. This position forces us to consider new approaches to establishing subject homogeneity in clinical studies, such as selecting individuals with a positive family history for Tourette's syndrome and tics, *vs* patients with a negative family history, or haloperidol responders *vs* nonresponders. Despite our increasing knowledge of central nervous system neuropharmacology, we continue to practice a *black box* pharmacotherapy with TS. Our therapeutic approaches are empirical; our neurochemical investigations follow these initial trial-and-error leads. Future investigations of TS will require both clinical sophistication and neurochemical technology if we are to understand thoroughly the genesis of this disorder.

REFERENCES

1. Eldridge R, Sweet R, Lake CR, et al: Gilles de la Tourette's syndrome: Clinical, genetic, psychologic, and biochemical aspects in 21 selected families. *Neurology (Minneap)* 27:115–124, 1977.
2. Eldridge R, Wassman ER, Nee L, et al: Gilles de la Tourette syndrome, in Goodman RM, Motielsky AG (eds): *Diseases Among Ashkenazi Jews.* New York, Raven Press, 1979, pp 171–185.
3. Wilson RS, Garron DC, Klawans HL: Significance of genetic factors in Gilles de la Tourette syndrome: A review. *Behav Genet* 8:503–510, 1978.
4. Nee LE, Caine ED, Polinsky RJ, et al: Gilles de la Tourette syndrome: Clinical and family study of 50 cases. *Ann Neurol* 7:41–49, 1980.
5. Shapiro AK, Shapiro ES, Bruun RD, et al: *Gilles de la Tourette Syndrome.* New York, Raven Press, 1978.
6. Mendelson WB, Caine ED, Goyer P, et al: Sleep in Gilles de la Tourette syndrome. *Biol Psychiat* 15:339–343, 1980.
7. Caine ED, Margolin DI, Brown GL, et al: Gilles de la Tourette's syndrome, tardive dyskinesia, and psychosis in an adolescent. *Am J Psychiatry* 135: 241–243, 1978.
8. Caine ED, Polinsky RJ: Tardive dyskinesia in persons with Gilles de la Tourette's disease. *Arch Neurol,* 38:471–472, 1981.
9. Caine ED, Polinsky RJ: Haloperidol-induced dysphoria in patients with Tourette syndrome. *Am J Psychiatry* 136:1216–1217, 1979.
10. Van Putten T, May PRA: "Akinetic" depression in schizophrenia. *Arch Gen Psychiatry* 35:1101–1107, 1978.

11. Caine ED, Mendelson WB, Loriaux DL: Neuroendocrine effects of haloperidol in an adolescent with Gilles de la Tourette's disease and delayed onset of puberty. *J Nerv Ment Dis* 167:504–507, 1979.

12. Caine ED, Polinsky RJ, Kartzinel R, et al: The trial use of clozapine for abnormal involuntary movement disorders. *Am J Psychiatry* 136:317–320, 1979.

13. Carlsson A, Corrodi H, Fuxe K, et al: Effect of antidepressant drugs on the depletion of intraneuronal brain 5-hydroxytryptamine stores caused by 4-methyl-gamma-ethyl, meta-tyramine. *Eur J Pharmacol* 5:357–366, 1969.

14. Asberg M, Ringberger V, Sjoqvist F, et al: Monoamine metabolites in cerebrospinal fluid and serotonin uptake inhibition during treatment with chlorimipramine. *Clin Pharmacol Ther* 21:201–207, 1977.

15. Carlsson A, Corrodi H, Fuxe K, et al: Effects of some antidepressant drugs on the depletion of intraneuronal brain catecholamine stores caused by 4-gamma-dimethyl-meta-tyramine. *Eur J Pharmacol* 5:367–373, 1969.

16. Yaryura-Tobias JA, Neziroglu FA: Gilles de la Tourette syndrome: A new clinico-therapeutic approach. *Prog Neuropsychopharmacol* 1:335–338, 1977.

17. Caine ED, Polinsky RJ, Ebert MH, et al: Trial of chlorimipramine and desipramine for Gilles de la Tourette syndrome. *Ann Neurol* 5:305–306, 1979.

18. Polinsky RJ, Ebert MH, Caine ED, et al: Cholinergic treatment in the Tourette syndrome. *N Engl J Med* 302:1310, 1980.

11 New Horizons in the Treatment of Neuropsychiatric Disorders

Richard L. Borison
Anthony J. Blowers
Bruce I. Diamond

In discussing the treatment of neuropsychiatric disorders, and particularly tardive dyskinesia, one has to have some idea of how these occur and how to avoid them. Many different drugs have been used in efforts to treat tardive dyskinesia when it occurs (see Chapters 8, 12, and 13), but when it occurs it is already too late. Therefore, one should be thinking first of how to avoid it. The easiest way to approach the subject is to review the neuropharmacology of the striatum or extrapyramidal system (see Chapter 1 for a more detailed review), and this can be simplified by looking only at the midbrain, substantia nigra, which sends nerve fibers to the striatum, the caudate and putamen nuclei. These nerve fibers release dopamine as the neurotransmitter and then communicate or synapse with neurons that are intrinsic to the striatum. These striatal neurons release acetylcholine as the neurotransmitter. Finally, there is a feedback loop from the striatum to the substantia nigra and these nerve fibers release GABA as the neurotransmitter. It is very important to note what these different neurotransmitters do in the brain, because this helps in understanding the rationale for treating extrapyramidal movement disorders. Dopamine has an inhibitory effect, while acetylcholine is facilitating, and the entire pharmacology of the extrapyramidal system can be understood as a balance between the inhibitory effects of dopamine and the facilitating effects of acetylcholine. They are in balance in a normally functioning extrapyramidal system.

In order to discuss the drug-induced movement disorders, it is instructive to first look at some experiments in nature. One such experiment in nature is idiopathic Parkinson's disease. In Parkinson's disease there is a degeneration and a loss of dopamine-containing nerve fibers. The dopamine input is lost and the balance is tipped in favor of acetylcholine, so that in idiopathic Parkinson's disease there is too much acetylcholine and too little dopamine. Another experiment in nature is Huntington's chorea, which is an inherited movement disorder characterized by hyperkinesias, or too much movement. In the brains of patients with Huntington's chorea there is a degeneration of the GABA-containing nerve pathway and a degeneration of the acetylcholine-containing nerve pathway; acetylcholine and GABA are diminished while the dopamine pathway is left intact, which shifts the balance in favor of dopamine and produces a preponderance of dopamine effects and a deficit of acetylcholine effects. This is all the information one needs to know to understand drug-induced movement disorders and the rationale for their treatments.

The drug-induced extrapyramidal side effects (EPS) commonly seen in psychiatric patients include: akathisia, dystonia, drug-induced parkinsonism, and tardive dyskinesia. Before discussing tardive dyskinesia, it may be helpful to review some of these other, acutely occurring, extrapyramidal side effects, as this can facilitate the understanding of tardive dyskinesia. The dystonias, or dystonic reactions, are usually recognized as a clonic or fixed contraction of a group of muscles. The neck usually is involved causing a torticollis or retrocollis, or the eye muscles are involved and the eyes roll back in the head, the so-called oculogyric crisis. Occasionally the laryngeal muscles can be involved and patients develop a laryngospasm which potentially can be life threatening. This is often misdiagnosed as an allergic reaction to the medication, but it is a laryngospasm, a dystonic reaction involving the laryngeal muscles. Younger patients are more susceptible, and male patients are more susceptible than female patients to dystonic reactions. These usually occur early, within 48 to 72 hours of initiating treatment or increasing the dose of the antipsychotic drug. Dystonic reactions are treated with anticholinergic drugs, ie, benztropine (Cogentin), trihexyphenidyl (Artane), and procyclidine (Kemedrin). The anticholinergic drugs work in the treatment of acute dystonic reactions because the normal balance of the extrapyramidal system is disturbed by the antipsychotic drug in favor of acetylcholine. That imbalance can be restored to normal balance by giving anticholinergic drugs to diminish the acetylcholine input and placing it into balance with the reduced dopamine input, thus reversing the dystonic reaction.

It is important to realize that there is a rationale for why these drugs work and that they are not used simply because they work; they are used because there is a reason for why they work. Diphenhydramine (Benadryl), an antihistamine, has a very high index of anticholinergic activity, and it is probably the anticholinergic activity of diphenhydramine that works like trihexyphenidyl and benztropine to reverse the dystonic reactions. Drugs that increase dopamine input, such as amphetamines, and levodopa, could be used to treat dystonic reactions but these drugs are not selective. They increase the dopamine input in the extrapyramidal system but can also increase it in the limbic system, so when levodopa or amphetamine is given to schizophrenic patients they can become more psychotic and, for this reason, these drugs usually are not used to treat drug-induced dystonic reactions. A very interesting aspect of dystonia musculorum deformans, an idiopathic illness in which patients spontaneously develop dystonic reactions — usually torsion dystonias — is that it has the same pharmacology (see Chapter 5). One of the most effective drugs used in the treatment of dystonia musculorum deformans is levodopa, and it does not make these nonpsychotic individuals psychotic.

Amantadine increases the release and blocks the reuptake of dopamine. So amantadine (Symmetrel) increases dopamine input and restores a normal balance in patients with neuroleptic-induced EPS. It also seems to have a selective effect on the extrapyramidal system. Some patients with renal failure or poor renal function will develop toxic levels of amantadine because this drug is excreted by the kidneys unmetabolized. When that happens, the amantadine effect will spill over to the limbic system and patients can become psychotic. But, in general, amantadine has a selective effect on the extrapyramidal system.

Barbiturates can reverse EPS by producing sedation. Every extrapyramidal movement disorder, with one exception, disappears during sleep. The exception is ballismus or hemiballismus, where patients have the ballistic or throwing movements of the limbs, which do not disappear during sleep (see Chapter 5). The involuntary movements of Parkinson's disease, drug-induced parkinsonism, Tourette's syndrome, tardive dyskinesia, and Huntington's chorea, all disappear during sleep. Barbiturates may reverse dystonic reactions by inducing sedation but they also decrease the release of acetylcholine. And if they decrease the release of acetylcholine, they will restore the normal balance, so barbiturates can also reverse dystonic reactions because of their effects on acetylcholine.

Caffeine impedes the absorption of antipsychotic drugs from the stomach into the blood stream, so giving caffeine will result in less drug reaching the brain, thereby avoiding dystonic reactions. But a patient with an acute dystonic reaction already has enough drug in the brain so that giving caffeine will not reverse the reaction by impeding absorption of the drug. Caffeine has another mechanism of action, however, and this is why it helps in drug-induced EPS. When dopamine receptors are stimulated in the extrapyramidal system this sets off a chain of reactions, which ultimately realize themselves by increasing the levels of cyclic adenosine monophosphate (AMP). Caffeine blocks the breakdown of cyclic AMP, which increases levels of cyclic AMP and, thus, caffeine can potentiate dopamine effects. So when caffeine is given to a patient with drug-induced EPS it is in essence increasing the dopamine input and restoring the normal balance again.

Neurologists will usually describe the four cardinal signs of parkinsonism as: 1) rigidity, 2) loss of postural reflexes, 3) tremor, and 4) akinesia. Parkinsonian tremor is a resting tremor, and not an action or postural tremor. It is important to make this differentiation because other drugs can produce action tremors. Lithium and alcohol produce an action or postural tremor. The best treatment for action or postural tremor is propranolol, which does not work very well in parkinsonian tremor. Sometimes when a patient is shaky all over it is difficult to know whether it is a resting or an action tremor. A very easy way to make the differentiation is have the patient sit in a chair with his hands in his lap. He might even have the tremor at rest. Then have him reach up and touch your finger. If, as he reaches up to touch your finger, the tremor tends to diminish, it is a resting tremor. If, as he tries to touch your finger, the tremor increases, that is an action tremor. Resting tremors do not respond to propranolol (Inderal) while action tremors do. Other types of action tremors, such as benign familial, or essential tremor, also respond to propranolol treatment.

Rigidity has to do with a change in muscle tone and thus is detected by taking the patient's arm or another joint and putting that joint through a passive range of movements. If you can feel the so-called cogwheel rigidity, the little give and take — it feels like cogs fitting into a wheel — then rigidity can be diagnosed. Akinesia or bradykinesia is a lack of movement or a slowing of initiation of movement. Sometimes when treating with antipsychotic drugs something resembling catatonic schizophrenia is seen, when what has actually happened is that the patient has become akinetic. He is not moving very much, sometimes with a somewhat flexed posture (perhaps a waxy flexibility). Antipsychotic drugs can produce akinesia, a slowness of movement. Therefore, if a patient appears to suddenly develop catatonic schizophrenia during antipsychotic drug treatment, he probably became akinetic as a result of medication.

Another sign of parkinsonism is the mask-like face; the facial muscles are bradykinetic and rigid so the patient tends to have a rather fixed, expressionless face. Drooling is seen in parkinsonian patients, not because they produce too much saliva, but because they cannot swallow. The extrapyramidal system controls the act of deglutition, and when the involved muscles become rigid and bradykinetic, patients have difficulty swallowing. Beyond the aesthetic concern, this drooling has clinical significance because these patients are at great risk for aspirating fluid.

Postural reflexes are also impaired in patients with Parkinson's disease or drug-induced parkinsonism, and this manifests as a shift in the center of gravity. Under normal conditions while standing, the trunk is aligned with the legs so that the center of gravity is where the feet are. This shifts in parkinsonism so that the center of gravity tends to be in front of the patient. These patients have a somewhat stooped posture and they often have a characteristically narrow-based, shuffling gait. Sometimes patients have loss of postural reflexes without postural and gait disturbances and it is important to recognize this also. The easiest way to identify this is to have the patient sit down. A person with normal postural reflexes will know where his body is in space when he sits down. With loss of postural reflexes, the patient tries to sit down but will fall down into the chair. Arising from the chair becomes difficult for these patients, partly due to bradykinesia but also due to loss of postural reflexes. The patient has difficulty getting up and then when on his feet, he has a tendency to fall forward or to lose his balance. Another test for loss of postural reflexes is to have the patient stand and then to have the examiner disrupt his balance by giving him a small push. The normal person, when pushed, will regain his balance, but in the parkinsonian patient with loss of postural reflexes, just a small push will cause the patient to fall backward. Loss of postural reflexes can be very important. In a parkinsonian patient, just a little push, an accidental bump, or a difficult maneuver on an icy pathway may cause him to fall down and possibly break a hip or other bones. Drug-induced parkinsonism can occur without tremor, but since the tremor is usually the last thing to occur, a patient may develop this disorder without ever having tremor.

Akathisia is the inability to stay still or motor restlessness. Patients will often pace back and forth and say, "Well, my legs feel nervous, my knees feel jumpy." By strict definition, however, akathisia is a subjective feeling of restlessness and when it becomes severe it spills over into the motor sphere and restless movement is noticed. It is important to listen carefully to the complaints of patients taking antipsychotic drugs who will often say, "I feel all nervous and uptight inside." The clinician sometimes naively concludes that he has treated the psychosis and uncovered an underlying neurotic conflict with anxiety for which he then prescribes diazepam (Valium). And when the diazepam appears to relieve the anxiety, his conclusion is reaffirmed. It is important to remember, however, that diazepam works through the GABA system and by this mechanism it may be helpful to patients with akathisia. Therefore, patients taking antipsychotic drugs who complain about being nervous or uptight may have akathisia rather than an anxiety disorder. Akathisia is probably the most drug-resistant, acutely occurring extrapyamidal side effect. Diazepam, anticholinergic drugs, or amantadine will not help every patient and, frequently, the only way to treat akathisia is either to decrease the dose of the antipsychotic drug, which will reestablish the dopamine input, or to give an antipsychotic drug that is less likely to cause EPS.

Dyskinesias are abnormal involuntary muscular movements. In tardive dyskinesia choreoathetoid movements are usually seen, often involving the facial-lingual-buccal muscles. Sometimes the extremities or the trunk are involved, and at times the diaphragm is also involved with patients developing respiratory alkalosis. Laryngeal muscles can be involved and patients can have difficulty swallowing. Dyskinesias are abnormal involuntary muscular movements. Tardive is from the word tardy or late, implying that these are late occurring, abnormal involuntary muscular movements. Tardive dyskinesia is iatrogenic, and it is difficult for most physicians to admit that they produce tardive dyskinesia in patients. Many people will point out that Bleuler described dyskinesias in patients before antipsychotic drugs were used, and that tardive dyskinesia might be something that occurs naturally as a part of schizophrenia. It is more likely that Bleuler was describing patients with Huntington's chorea, Tourette's syndrome, or senile choreas. Studies have shown, in comparing patients with spontaneous choreas to patients with chorea and a past history of antipsychotic drug treatment, there is a fortyfold greater incidence in those who received antipsychotics. Clearly then, iatrogenic chorea is a common result of treatment with antipsychotic drugs.

Descriptively, the drug-induced dyskinesias can be separated into three distinct types: withdrawal dyskinesia, tardive dyskinesia, and covert dyskinesia. Withdrawal dyskinesias are acutely occurring dyskinesias, which are seen when the dose of drug is either stopped or withdrawn. They are, by definition, reversible but this may take up to 9 to 12 months. Tardive dyskinesias are irreversible or persistent. Covert dyskinesias are those that are masked by the antipsychotic drug, so they are not actually seen, but this is like sweeping dirt under the carpet. In a recent study, we lowered the dose of antipsychotic drug in ten randomly chosen patients and eight out of the ten developed dyskinesias. They had covert dyskinesias, which were uncovered by reducing drug dosage. That could be important because if it is known that a patient develops tardive dyskinesia when antipsychotic drug dosage is reduced, it means that at some point there was a covert dyskinesia. And if the dyskinesia was not looked for, it would certainly have been missed.

How does one look for covert dyskinesias? One way is to lower the dose of the antipsychotic drug, or to give an anticholinergic drug like trihexyphenidyl or benztropine, which may shift the balance enough to uncover covert dyskinesias (see Chapters 1 and 14). Thioridazine (Mellaril), of all the antipsychotic drugs currently marketed, appears to produce very little tardive dyskinesia. Gerlach and Simmelsgaard[1] described 16 patients with tardive dyskinesia in whom they discontinued all medications and evaluated the patients' involuntary movements with a rating scale. They then put them on thioridazine for four months. At the end of four months, the drug was discontinued, with a four-week wash-out. The tardive dyskinesia then was reassessed and the findings showed the disorder had not progressed. Since tardive dyskinesia is thought to be irreversible, nothing would have been expected to reverse it, but the thioridazine did not make it progress. They then took the same 16 patients and gave them 5.25 mg daily of haloperidol (Haldol), which masked the dyskinesia. After stopping the haloperidol, the dyskinesia was found to have progressed. They then questioned whether haloperidol, in combination with an anticholinergic drug, benztropine, might have the same effect as giving thioridazine alone. As might be expected, when they reassessed the tardive dyskinesia after this treatment combination it had progressed. Thus, there does not appear to be a relationship between the anticholinergic properties of thioridazine and its decreased propensity to cause tardive dyskinesia.

Although the central nervous system (CNS) is unique in its complexities, it shares many common properties with the peripheral nervous system (PNS) including the potential to develop denervation hypersensitivity. In fact, the recognition of this phenomenon in the peripheral nervous system led to the application of this concept to CNS function, and this is currently the most widely accepted hypothesis for tardive dyskinesia[2] (see Chapter 1). Another area in which the PNS may serve as a model for the CNS, is in the understanding of receptor differentiation and site specificity. Examples of receptor differentiation in the PNS include muscarinic and nicotinic cholinergic receptors, as well as alpha (α) and beta (β) noradrenergic receptors. An example of site specificity is the difference between β-receptors in the heart (β_1) and lung (β_2) and their different pharmacologies. Although these concepts are recognized scientifically and clinically in the PNS, their parallels in the CNS, particularly with respect to dopamine receptors, have been largely ignored.

Electrophysiological studies in the cat striatum have demonstrated that dopamine may have both excitatory and inhibitory actions on cell firing,[3] and similar results have been obtained in other species.[4] Moreover, these two populations of dopamine receptors appear to have different pharmacologies,[5] and can be further distinguished by their behavioral pharmacologies.[6] Behavioral studies have also led to a differentiation between dopamine receptors, separating them by their ability to produce either behavioral depression or activation. The dopamine receptors that produce behavioral depression have been termed autoreceptors.[7] These autoreceptors are presynaptic in origin and possess a greater affinity for dopamine than do the postsynaptic receptors.[8] Moreover, clinical studies involving the administration of dopamine agonists to patients with schizophrenia or tardive dyskinesia confirm the existence of two separate and antagonistic types of dopamine receptors with differing affinities for dopamine.[9,10] Biochemical evidence has established that the presynaptic striatal dopamine receptor (autoreceptor) regulates the biosynthesis of dopamine[11,12]; however, in the nigrostriatal system there is a third dopamine receptor type in the substantia nigra, which also regulates dopamine biosynthesis and can be pharmacologically distinguished from the presynaptic autoreceptor.[13]

The most systematic attempt at differentiating between dopamine receptor types has classified them according to whether or not they are coupled to adenylate cyclase.[14] It has been demonstrated that the limbic and striatal systems each contain dopamine receptors of both types: those which are coupled to adenylate cyclase (D_1) and those which are not (D_2); whereas, the tuberoinfundibular system is unique in possessing no D_1 presynaptic dopamine receptors, but only D_2 postsynaptic receptors.[15] Further evidence for discrete and distinguishable dopamine receptors comes from receptor-binding studies, which distinguish a high and a low affinity receptor type.[16,17] Other evidence suggests that dopamine receptors in the brain may be different in disease states such as schizophrenia.[18,19] Along these lines, it has been demonstrated that thioridazine best blocks those dopamine receptors which have been sensitized,[20] suggesting a mechanism of action for its clinical antipsychotic properties.

Biochemical studies have also elucidated pharmacological differences among dopamine receptors according to their location in the brain (site specificity). Most neuroleptics block dopamine receptors in both the striatum and mesolimbic system, producing a compensatory increase in dopamine turnover. There are, however, certain atypical antipsychotic agents (eg, clozapine, thioridazine, and sulpiride), which cause a much greater turnover of dopamine in the limbic compared with the extrapyramidal system, an action which is not accounted for by the anticholinergic activity of these drugs.[21,22] This evidence has been linked to a brain site specificity of action for these drugs, and these findings from animal studies correlate with the clinically observed lack of extrapyramidal side effects associated with these atypical neuroleptics.

In order to better demonstrate a site-specific action for various antipsychotic agents, we have conducted both human and animal studies. If atypical neuroleptic agents truly have a specific action on limbic rather than striatal dopamine receptors, they should then be unable to produce the striatal dopamine receptor denervation hypersensitivity that occurs secondary to receptor blockade (see Chapter 1). To test this hypothesis, white male Sprague-Dawley rats were used in an animal paradigm for tardive dyskinesia.[23] In this model, animals received daily administration of an antipsychotic drug during a three week period, after which the animals then received daily saline injections over five days. To assess dopamine receptor sensitization, the animals were challenged with the direct-acting dopamine agonist, apomorphine, in a dose which fails to produce a behavioral response in control animals. In our studies, we found that thioridazine produced a short-lived sensitization of striatal dopamine receptors (Figure 11-1), whereas haloperidol (Figure 11-2) and fluphenazine (Figure 11-3) produced more marked and longer-lived receptor sensitization. Other animal studies, in particular primate studies,[24,25] have also demonstrated dyskinetogenic (dopamine receptor hypersensitivity induction) potential, and have also found agents such as haloperidol to be much more potent in inducing this phenomenon.

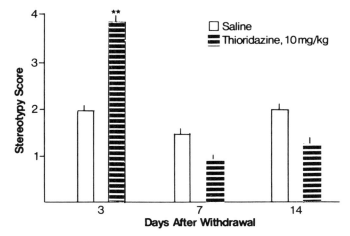

Figure 11-1 Apomorphine-induced stereotypy in rats after chronic thioridazine.

140

If atypical antipsychotic agents produce less dyskinesia in animals, may they then be less likely to produce dyskinesias in man? To test this hypothesis, one of us (AJB) conducted a survey of 309 patients in British geriatric centers. The mean age of our study group was 82.4 years. Patients were rated for dyskinesias by using a modified Abnormal Involuntary Movement Scale[26] (see Appendix II) and the Abbreviated

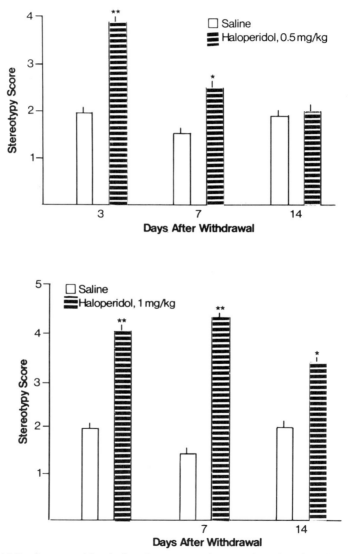

Figure 11-2 Apomorphine-induced stereotypy in rats after chronic haloperidol.

Dyskinesia Rating Scale of the Rockland Research Institute.[27] It was found that 48% of patients receiving antipsychotic drug treatment showed demonstrable dyskinesias. The incidence of dyskinesia was least with thioridazine treatment, and the severity of dyskinesias was greatest with conventional neuroleptic agents (Figure 11-4). This study extends our previous report,[28] which demonstrated a lower incidence and severity of tardive dyskinesia in patients receiving thioridazine as compared to those receiving haloperidol (see also Chapter 14). Similarly, it was also shown that clozapine and thioridazine are less likely then haloperidol to make a preexisting tardive dyskinesia progress.[29] This also implies that atypical antipsychotics may be less likely to produce dyskinesias in man.[29-31] If this is true, it must be questioned as to what unique properties of the atypical antipsychotic agents render them less dyskinetogenic. This difference in the potential to produce dyskinesia might be accounted for by the findings from animal studies that demonstrate a site specificity of action in brain for atypical antipsychotics. We have now tested this hypothesis in man.

Human brain material was collected within six hours of death and, with the aid of a neuropathologist, areas from the limbic system (olfactory tubercle, nucleus accumbens) and extrapyramidal system (caudate nucleus, putamen) were dissected. Tissues were homogenized and prepared in a sodium-potassium-phosphate buffer. Receptor ligand binding was carried out using ^{3}H-spiroperidol[32] and specific binding was ascertained using (+)-butaclamol. It was found that the high affinity

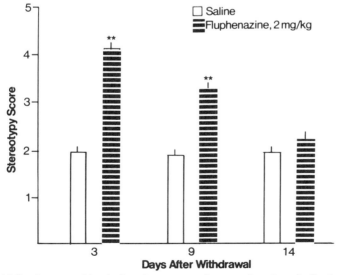

Figure 11-3 Apomorphine-induced stereotypy in rats after chronic fluphenazine.

142

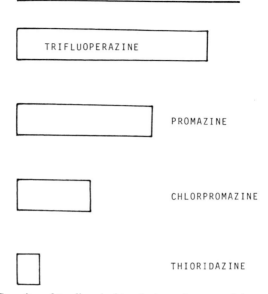

Figure 11-4 Severity of tardive dyskinesia in patients receiving trifluoperazine, promazine, chlorpromazine, and thioridazine.

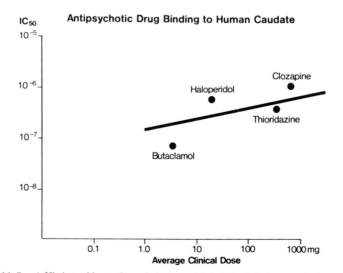

Figure 11-5 Affinity of butaclamol, haloperidol, thioridazine, and clozapine for striatal dopamine receptors.

dopamine receptor site showed a $K_D = 0.8$ nM. Using striatal tissue, haloperidol and butaclamol were the most potent in displacing the tritiated ligand, whereas clozapine and thioridazine were several orders of magnitude less potent (Figure 11-5). In contrast, all four neuroleptics were within the same order of magnitude in their abilities to block limbic dopamine receptors (Figure 11-6). Interestingly, prochlorperazine (Compazine), an antiemetic drug that produces a high incidence of EPS, has a high affinity for extrapyramidal dopamine receptors but a low affinity for limbic dopamine receptors, which may account for the very weak antipsychotic properties of this drug.

In comparing receptor blockade in the limbic rather than extrapyramidal system (Figure 11-7), clozapine and thioridazine clearly showed a site specificity for blocking limbic dopamine receptors. This site specificity may therefore account for the relative paucity of acute and chronic EPS observed in patients treated with thioridazine or clozapine, and may explain why these two drugs produce less tardive dyskinesia than is seen with the other neuroleptic drugs, which are more likely to block striatal rather than limbic dopamine receptors.

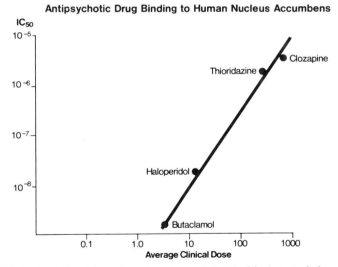

Figure 11-6 Affinity of butaclamol, haloperidol, thioridazine, and clozapine for limbic dopamine receptors.

144

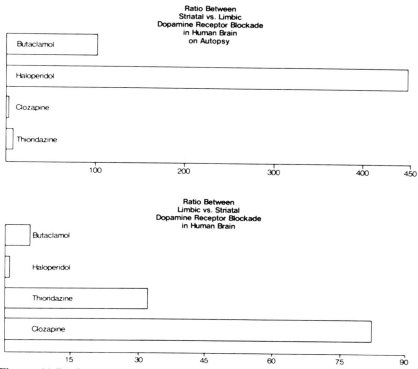

Figure 11-7 Comparison of relative affinities of butaclamol, haloperidol, thioridazine, and clozapine for human striatal and limbic dopamine receptors.

REFERENCES

1. Gerlach J, Simmelsgaard H: Tardive dyskinesia during and following treatment with haloperidol, haloperidol + biperiden, thioridazine, and clozapine. *Psychopharmacology* 59:105–112, 1978.

2. Klawans HL: The pharmacology of tardive dyskinesia. *Am J Psychiatry* 130:82–86, 1973.

3. York DH: Possible dopaminergic pathway from substantia nigra to putamen. *Brain Res* 20:233–249, 1970.

4. Cools AR, van Rossum JM: Excitation-mediating and inhibition-mediating dopamine receptors: A new concept towards a better understanding of electrophysiological, biochemical, pharmacological, functional and clinical data. *Psychopharmacologia* 45:243–254, 1976.

5. Struyker Boudier HAJ, Gielen W, Cools AR, et al: Pharmacological analysis of dopamine-induced inhibition and excitation of neurons of the snail *helix aspersa*. *Arch Int Pharmacodyn* 209:324–331, 1974.

6. Cools AR: Two functionally and pharmacologically distinct dopamine receptors in the rat brain. *Adv Biochem Psychopharmacology* 16:215–225, 1977.

145

7. Carlsson A: Some aspects of dopamine in the basal ganglia, in Yahr MD (ed): *The Basal Ganglia*. New York, Raven Press, 1976, pp 181–189.

8. Strombom U: Catecholamine receptor agonists: Effects on motor activity and rate of tyrosine hydroxylation in mouse brain. *Naunyn Schmiedeberg's Arch Pharmacol* 292:167–176, 1976.

9. Smith RC, Tamminga CA, Haraszti J, et al: Effects of dopamine agonists in tardive dyskinesia. *Am J Psychiatry* 134:763–768, 1977.

10. Carroll BJ, Curtis GC, Kokmen E: Paradoxical response to dopamine agonists in tardive dyskinesia. *Am J Psychiatry* 134:785–789, 1977.

11. DiChiara G, Porceddu ML, Fratta W, et al: Postsynaptic receptors are not essential for dopaminergic feedback regulation. *Nature* 267:270–272, 1977.

12. Roth RH: Dopamine autoreceptors: Pharmacology, function, and comparison with post-synaptic dopamine receptors. *Commun Psychopharmacol* 3:429–445, 1979.

13. Groppetti A, Parenti M, Cattabeni F, et al: Dopaminergic receptor activity in substantia nigra in the mechanism of autoregulation of striatal dopamine release. *Adv Biochem Psychopharmacology* 19:363–372, 1978.

14. Kebabian JW, Calne DB: Multiple receptors for dopamine. *Nature* 277:93–96, 1979.

15. Costa E, Gessa GL: *Non-striatal Dopaminergic Neurons*. New York, Raven Press, 1977.

16. Pedigo NW, Reisine TD, Fields JZ, et al: ³H-spiroperidol binding to two receptor sites in both the corpus striatum and frontal cortex of rat brain. *Eur J Pharmacology* 50:451–453, 1978.

17. Andorn AC, Maguire ME: ³H-spiroperidol binding in rat striatum: two high-affinity sites of differing selectivities. *J Neurochemistry* 35:1105–1113, 1980.

18. Lee T, Seeman P, Touretellotte WW, et al: Binding of ³H-neuroleptics and ³H-apomorphine in schizophrenic brains. *Nature* 274:897–900, 1978.

19. Owen F, Crow TJ, Poulter M, et al: Increased dopamine-receptor sensitivity in schizophrenia. *Lancet* 2:223–225, 1978.

20. Diamond BI, Borison RL: Behavioral effects of intralimbic phenothiazine administration to rats, in Usdin E, Eckert H, Forrest IS (eds): *Phenothiazines and Structurally Related Compounds: Basic and Clinical Studies*. New York, Elsevier, 1980, pp 269–272.

21. Bowers MB, Rozitis A: Regional differences in homovanillic acid concentrations after acute and chronic administration of antipsychotic drugs. *J Pharm Pharmacol* 26:743–745, 1974.

22. Crow TJ, Deaken JFW, Johnstone EC, et al: Dopamine and schizophrenia. *Lancet* 2:563–566, 1976.

23. Tarsy D, Baldessarini RJ: Behavioural supersensitivity to apomorphine following chronic treatment with drugs which interfere with the synaptic function of catecholamines. *Neuropharmacology* 13:927–940, 1974.

24. Gunne LM, Barany S: A monitoring test for the liability of neuroleptic drugs to induce tardive dyskinesia. *Psychopharmacology* 63:195–198, 1979.

25. Liebman J, Neale R: Neuroleptic-induced acute dyskinesias in squirrel monkeys: Correlation with propensity to cause extrapyramidal side effects. *Psychopharmacology* 68:25–29, 1980.

26. Development of a dyskinetic movement scale, *National Institute of Mental Health Psychopharmacology Research Branch Publication* #4, 1975, pp 3–6.

27. Simpson GM, Lee JH, Zoubok B, et al: A rating scale for tardive dyskinesia. *Psychopharmacology* 64:171–179, 1979.

28. Blowers AJ, Bicknell J: The relevance of antipsychotic medication in tardive dyskinesia in the elderly, in Usdin E, Eckert H, Forrest IS (eds): *Phenothiazines and Structurally Related Compounds: Basic and Clinical Studies.* New York, Elsevier, 1980, pp 337–340.

29. Gerlach J: Tardive dyskinesia. *Dan Med Bull* 26:209–245, 1979.

30. *American Psychiatric Association: Tardive Dyskinesia.* Task force report #18. American Psychiatric Association, Washington, DC, 1980.

31. Klawans HL, Goetz CG, Perlik S: Tardive dyskinesia: Review and update. *Am J Psychiatry* 137:900–908, 1980.

32. Fields JZ, Reisine TD, Yamamura HI: Biochemical demonstration of dopaminergic receptors in rat and human brain using ^{3}H spiroperidol. *Brain Res* 136:578–584, 1977.

12 A Treatment Approach Directed Toward Decreasing Receptor Sensitivity

Murray Alpert
Arnold J. Friedhoff

Increase in dopamine receptor sensitivity is generally thought to underlie tardive dyskinesia (TD). The increased sensitivity is thought to result from decreased access of dopamine to the postsynaptic receptors through the blocking action of neuroleptic drugs. We have been studying a novel treatment approach to TD, testing the hypothesis that dopamine sensitivity can be down-regulated by temporarily increasing dopamine levels. To accomplish this, gradually increasing doses of levodopa are administered, continuing at each dose increment until evidence of adaptation is seen, and then increasing the dose until our target dose is reached. Following adaptation to the target dose, the levodopa is discontinued. It is expected that improvement will persist if normal receptor sensitivity is reestablished and transmitter levels are permitted to return to their usual levels.

Workers in our group have modeled these processes in animal studies.[1] They have shown that rats exposed to neuroleptics show increase in the number and activity of dopamine receptors and that subsequent exposure to levodopa can return receptor number and activity to baseline levels. This is a report of clinical dose ranging studies as we attempt to define optimal parameters of this treatment for patients with tardive dyskinesia.

Our dependent measure is the Abnormal Involuntary Movement Scale (AIMS) administered as recommended by the Psychopharmacology Research Branch of NIMH[2] (see Appendix II).

Subjects

For inclusion in our study patients are required to have scores of at least mildly severe (2 points) on the lips, jaws, and tongue (items 2, 3 and 4) or moderately severe (3 points) on items 2 or 3 or 4. Patients are eliminated from the study when there is evidence of abnormal involuntary movements prior to exposure to neuroleptic drugs. Also required is at least a two-year exposure to neuroleptic drugs at reasonable clinical doses for inclusion in study. Patients with extensive limb and trunk movements are not excluded so long as they meet the above requirements. These criteria are designed to increase homogeneity and, hopefully, reproducibility of our findings.

Drugs

Initially our studies included only patients not on concurrent neuroleptic medications, more recently we have included such patients. In any case, all patients are followed during a baseline period of at least six weeks, during which time their neuroleptic medication is unchanged. Anticholinergic drugs are not permitted. Sedatives are permitted throughout the trial but not within twelve hours of a rating.

Procedures

In Figure 12-1, the treatment course is depicted. Inclusion criteria are evaluated at rating 1, baseline. At this point the patients' medications have been unchanged for at least six weeks. There is a four week "dose-finding" period, during which semi-weekly dose increments are attempted. Patients are randomly assigned to one of three doses: 30/300 mg/day, 50/500 mg/day, or 75/750 mg/day carbidopa/levodopa as Sinemet. Medication is administered in divided doses with meals.

The major factors limiting the rate of dose increase have been: 1) a

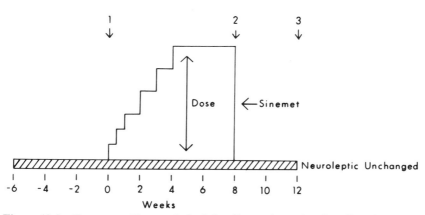

Figure 12-1 Treatment Course. 1, 2, & 3 reflect ratings. 1 = baseline; 2 = cut; 3 = termination. If patient is on concurrent neuroleptic medication, it is unchanged from weeks − 6 to + 12. Cut refers only to the experimental medication (Sinemet).

transient hypotension; 2) an increase in abnormal movements; 3) behavioral activation. Patients show tolerance in each of these areas, and dose increments are titrated against signs of adaptation. One patient showed a drug sensitivity (rash and skin flushing) to both Sinemet and levodopa, and one patient had a seizure, apparently unrelated to Sinemet, while on protocol. When used carefully, patients with TD, even if they are psychotic, can be managed on Sinemet with doses comparable to those used for akinesia.

Results

To date, 11 patients have been studied in the protocol shown in Figure 12-1. In Figure 12-2 only baseline and termination ratings are presented although evaluations were collected weekly. For comparison, data for ten patients who met the inclusion criteria and were evaluated on two occasions approximately 12 weeks apart are included. The comparison group was matched with the experimentals for age, sex, and baseline AIMS score. They did not, however, receive placebo.

In Figure 12-2 it can be seen that although there is a good deal of variability in terms of the response to treatment, patients in general showed some improvement and about half the patients showed a clinically significant change. This trend is not apparent in the comparison group. Improvement appeared similar for those treated with Sinemet in combination with neuroleptic as with Sinemet alone. There are not yet enough cases to examine for the effect of Sinemet dose.

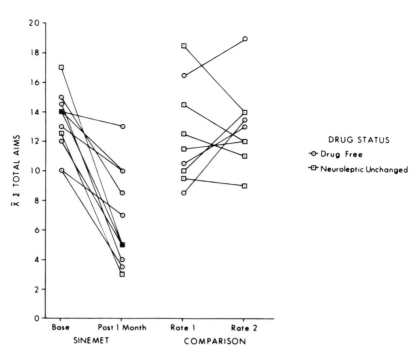

Figure 12-2 Abnormal movements of L-dopa treated (N = 11) and comparison group of equivalent baseline pathology (N = 10). Second rating (R2) is four months after baseline (R1).

In Figure 12-3 the group averages by AIMS area are presented for the experimental and comparison groups. Our inclusion criteria emphasized dyskinetic facial involvement and this is reflected in the baseline scores. The results are consistent with our clinical impression that oral area dyskinetic movements are more responsive to treatment than extremities where movements in both areas coexist.

The contrasts between the experimental and the comparison groups presented in Figures 12-2 and 12-3 were tested by analysis of covariance, and these results are presented in Table 12-1 where it can be seen that the difference in outcome between the two groups is statistically reliable. This comparison is not, of course, an appropriate test of the specific treatment since the comparison group did not receive placebo, or frequent ratings, or daily blood pressures, etc. However, the different dose groups were done in a double-blind manner, and it is hoped that when sufficient cases are collected, group differences may provide some evidence for efficacy. The results of this dose finding study will guide us in establishing treatment parameters for a straightforward double-blind outcome trial.

Table 12-1
Two-Way Analysis of Covariance AIMS

Groups: A1 = Sinemet treated (N = 10)
      A2 = Dyskinetics with no medication change (N = 15)

Total

Source	SS	DF	MS	F
Group (A)	78.75	1	78.75	12.12†
Sex (B)	4.45	1	4.45	.69
AB	13.45	1	13.45	2.07
Error within	149.40	23	6.50	

Facial Oral

Source	SS	DF	MS	F
Group (A)	34.11	1	34.11	5.25*
Sex (B)	.16	1	.16	.02
AB	6.01	1	6.01	.93
Error within	149.41	23	6.50	

Extremities

Source	SS	DF	MS	F
Group (A)	6.24	1	6.24	5.08*
Sex (B)	1.72	1	1.72	1.40
AB	.10	1	.10	.08
Error within	28.22	23	1.23	

*$p < 0.05$
†$p < 0.01$

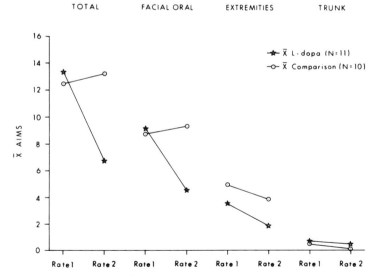

Figure 12-3 Abnormal movements of L-dopa treated (N = 11) and comparison group of equivalent baseline pathology (N = 10). Second rating (R2) is four months after baseline (R1).

DISCUSSION

A novel treatment approach to tardive dyskinesia has been described, based on the assumptions that it is related to an underlying pathogenic dopamine-receptor supersensitivity, and that this supersensitivity may be reversed if dopamine levels are increased. It has been shown that dopamine levels may be safely increased in psychotic dyskinetic patients if incremental steps are controlled carefully. When this is done there is some evidence that dyskinetic movements may be modestly exacerbated, initially. With adaptation to the levodopa, movements can be reduced while the medication is continued. When the medication is stopped, most patients show some reduction in dyskinetic movements. About half the patients show a marked improvement, which appears to be persisting for patients who can be maintained off neuroleptic drugs.

REFERENCES

1. Friedhoff AJ, Bonnet K, Rosengarten H: Reversal of two manifestations of dopamine receptor supersensitivity by administration of l-dopa. *Res Comm Chem Pathol Pharmacol* 16(3):411–423, 1977.
2. *ECDEU Assessment Manual for Psychopharmacology,* U.S. Department of Health, Education and Welfare, Revised, 1976.

13 Lecithin for the Treatment of Tardive Dyskinesia: Preliminary Results from a Double-Blind Study

Alan J. Gelenberg
Joanne D. Wojcik
John H. Growdon
Steven H. Zeisel
Richard J. Wurtman

The abnormal movements of tardive dyskinesia are believed to reflect an excess of dopamine vis-à-vis acetylcholine-mediated neurotransmission in the nigrostriatal pathway.[1] This imbalance, in turn, is thought to result from a denervation-type supersensitivity of postsynaptic dopamine receptors, brought about by long-term therapy with antipsychotic drugs. Therefore, approaches to the treatment of tardive dyskinesia have included attempts to decrease dopamine or increase acetylcholine activity[2] (see also Chapter 1).

One possible way to increase brain acetylcholine is via the oral administration of choline, the precursor of acetylcholine. In rats, oral choline administration has produced sequential elevations of blood choline, brain choline, and brain acetylcholine levels.[3,4] Davis et al administered choline chloride to a man with tardive dyskinesia and reported a decrease in his involuntary movements.[5] These investigators have since administered choline to a total of six patients and have found significant improvement in every case; however, three of the patients had no exacerbation of movements when placebo was substituted for choline, raising the question of spontaneous improvement.[6] Tamminga and associates administered choline to four patients with tardive dyskinesia: two improved, while the other two were prematurely terminated because of depressive symptoms.[7] Growdon and colleagues administered choline to 20 patients with tardive dyskinesia in a double-blind, placebo-controlled, crossover study.[8] Blood choline levels increased in every patient. By the second week of choline therapy, abnormal movements had decreased greatly in five patients, decreased moderately in four others, remained unchanged in ten, and appeared worse in one.

Most choline found in the normal diet is in the form of phosphatidylcholine, which consists of a glycerol molecule covalently bound to one molecule of phosphorylcholine and two molecules of fatty acids (Figure 13-1). Phosphatidylcholine, in turn, is contained in lecithin, a mixture of phosphorylated lipids, found in egg yolk, soy beans, fish and meat, legumes, and other foods. Lecithin is also used as an emulsifier in many processed foods.[9] In rats, the administration of a single meal rich in lecithin produces effects resembling those of choline: a sequential increase in blood choline, brain choline, and brain acetylcholine levels.[10] In man, oral lecithin administration has been shown to cause even greater and longer-lasting increases in serum choline levels than choline administration.[11]

In a non-blind pilot project, we were impressed that oral lecithin could produce favorable results in patients with tardive dyskinesia, comparable to those observed with choline chloride.[12] In addition, lecithin was associated with fewer unwanted effects than choline and was more acceptable to patients. Barbeau has reported similar results with lecithin

LECITHIN

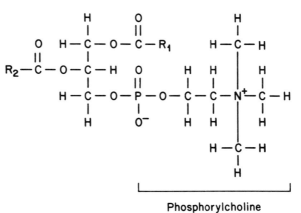

Phosphorylcholine

Figure 13-1 Structure of lecithin.

for the treatment of tardive dyskinesia.[13] Jackson et al found lecithin significantly more effective than placebo in suppressing the movements of tardive dyskinesia in every one of six patients studied.[14] In contrast to these positive impressions, Branchey and colleagues recently concluded that lecithin failed to produce improvement in eight chronic schizophrenic patients with tardive dyskinesia.[15] Their study differed from others in the literature in that they 1) used a different lecithin preparation (egg as opposed to soy), 2) employed a different treatment schedule (once-a-day, as opposed to three-times daily — and plasma choline levels do not appear to remain elevated on a once-daily schedule), and 3) did not measure plasma choline concentrations to determine whether dosage and compliance were adequate. Even so, their own data show that movement counts, in four of seven patients in whom they were recorded, were considerably lower during lecithin therapy than during placebo. In an average score of two eight-minute counts of movement frequency, one patient's decreased from 56.5 on placebo to 9 on lecithin, another's from 235.5 to 81.5, a third patient's from 130.5 to 22.5, while in a fourth movement frequency went from 27 to 0.

Because of the encouraging results to date with lecithin for the treatment of tardive dyskinesia, we have embarked on a double-blind, placebo-controlled, crossover study of outpatients with this disorder. This chapter will describe and discuss results from the first seven patients treated in this protocol.

METHODS

Patients

Patients were eligible for the study if they had a clinical diagnosis of tardive dyskinesia confirmed by both the project psychiatrist (AJG) and neurologist (JHG), based on the presence of choreoathetotic movements affecting the mouth, tongue, jaw, face, and/or extremities, which had begun in association with antipsychotic drug therapy. Attempts were made to exclude patients with other forms of extrapyramidal reactions, both naturally occurring and drug-induced, and schizophrenic mannerisms and stereotypies. The movements of tardive dyskinesia had to be present and stable for at least six months.

Procedure

Patients were treated as outpatients with lecithin and placebo for eight weeks each, separated by a two-week washout period, in a random-assignment crossover sequence. The dose of lecithin was 40 gm/day of a mixture containing 55% phosphatidylcholine. Because there is no acceptable placebo for lecithin at this time (this problem is currently being worked out), patients were instructed that they would receive two compounds of different lipid composition, one a solid (which actually contained the lecithin), the other a liquid (corn oil). They were instructed to mix a day's quantity of the substance in a blenderized emulsion at home, usually with milk and flavoring. The day's dose was then divided into three equal portions and taken on a three-times-daily schedule. No patient was receiving antiparkinson medication during the study. Other medications were held constant throughout the trial period.

Patients were rated every two weeks by a rater blind to which substance the patient was receiving. The rater did not discuss side effects with the patient. Rating instruments included the Abnormal Involuntary Movement Scale (AIMS) (see Appendix II), movement counts, and routine laboratory assessments. Serum concentrations of choline were measured by a radioenzymatic assay.

RESULTS

Seven patients have entered our study to date. Two patients were dropped within several days of entering the second treatment phase because of psychological decompensations; both had been assigned to placebo therapy in the first phase, so no data are available on their responses to lecithin. Data to be presented are based on the remaining five patients (Figure 13-2).

These five patients were all male, ranged in age from 32 to 45 years, and had had tardive dyskinesia of mild to moderate severity for two to six years. Psychiatric diagnoses were bipolar affective illness in two, chronic depression in two, and chronic schizophrenia in one. Concomitant medications, which were held constant throughout the study, included lithium carbonate, haloperidol, thioridazine, and diazepam.

Four of the five patients experienced some relief of movements during lecithin therapy that was greater than observed with placebo. The benefit tended to be partial and to affect some body parts more than others, but patients appreciated symptomatic relief and reported functional improvement. Moreover, movements returned to baseline levels in all of these cases when lecithin was withdrawn. In the fifth case, no change was seen with lecithin compared to placebo.

Based on mean values of the severity of abnormal movements, as measured by a total of AIMS items 1 through 7 at the end of each eight-week treatment period, placebo therapy was associated with a 10% im-

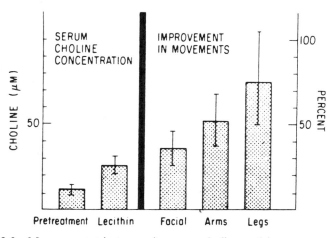

Figure 13-2 Mean percent increases in serum choline and improvement in abnormal movements in patients taking lecithin.

provement compared to baseline, while lecithin treatment was associated with a 26% improvement. The seven-item AIMS total averages were also computed comparing placebo and lecithin responses at the end of each two-week segment. At the end of the first two weeks, movements during lecithin were 28% worse than with placebo; by the end of week four, movements during lecithin were 1% better than during placebo, and this difference in favor of lecithin widened to 14% at the end of week six and to 21% by the end of week eight. Two patients received lecithin first, three received placebo first; the treatment sequence did not appear to make a difference. The number of patients in our study so far is too small to allow meaningful tests of statistical significance.

Adverse effects were relatively mild. Three patients experienced slight gastrointestinal upset. After the study, two patients were switched to a 100% phosphatidylcholine lecithin and developed parkinsonian signs; these remitted when the dose was lowered. The only mental status changes observed were improvement in those patients who showed a decrease in abnormal movements. Specifically, no patient showed depressive symptoms that worsened during lecithin treatment. No laboratory abnormalities were noted.

Plasma choline assays have been performed on three of the patients to date and demonstrate a roughly twofold increase in choline concentration during lecithin administration compared to baseline. Taking 40 gm/day of the 55% phosphatidylcholine lecithin, one patient's plasma choline concentration increased from 14.0 nmole/ml to 31.2, another's from 10.2 to 22.5. The third patient misunderstood our instructions to take the lecithin in three divided doses and was taking it only once daily at the time the plasma choline assay was performed. His plasma choline increased from 16.1 to 21.9. To date we have plasma choline assays on patients who have taken lecithin for up to four and one-half months continuously with no decrement in the elevated plasma choline concentration, suggesting that enzyme induction and pharmacokinetic tolerance do not occur over the period studied.

Plasma choline concentrations on one other patient are also worthy of note. This patient was being treated with lecithin in an attempt to suppress symptoms of mania. When he was not taking lecithin, plasma choline concentrations ranged between 10.6 and 13.8 nmole/ml. During therapy with 40 g/day of the 55% lecithin, choline concentrations increased to an average of 30.6. When the dose was raised to 60 g/day, plasma choline rose as high as 41.98, demonstrating a dose/response relationship.

DISCUSSION

Results from this limited patient sample support our earlier impression that lecithin can produce therapeutic benefit in patients suffering from tardive dyskinesia. Clinical improvement occurs gradually over one to two months. So far, in four of five patients with long-standing and persistent tardive dyskinesia, lecithin therapy was associated with a functional improvement not observed on placebo. When lecithin was withdrawn, movements worsened, which suggests that the improvement was a genuine drug effect, rather than a spontaneous remission. Also consistent with earlier impressions, adverse effects were minimal.

This patient sample needs to be expanded considerably before definitive conclusions can be reached about lecithin therapy for tardive dyskinesia. First, a statistically significant difference from placebo must be demonstrated. Second, it would be important to know what percentage of patients receive clinically meaningful benefit from lecithin. Then, it would be useful to identify possible predictors of response to therapy; we are about to use physostigmine tests for this purpose. In addition, if lecithin is effective, it would be important to establish a dose/response and/or plasma choline level/response relationship for this therapy.

Of all possible uses of dietary precursor therapy for neuropsychiatric disorders,[16,17] the use of choline and lecithin for the treatment of tardive dyskinesia has been the best studied to date and has produced the most clear-cut results. Tardive dyskinesia probably represents a better testing ground than diseases, such as Huntington's chorea and Alzheimer's dementia, which involve progressive neurologic deterioration, since in tardive dyskinesia the target population of brain neurons is presumably intact. However, the numbers of patients studied so far has been relatively few, and long term safety and efficacy of this treatment have yet to be definitively established.

An additional caveat is worth stating. When clinical investigators write about the use of "lecithin" for the treatment of disease states, they usually are referring to phosphatidylcholine. However, commercial lecithin, as is used in food processing and sold in health food stores, is defined as a mixture of phosphorylated lipids. The amount of phosphatidylcholine in lecithin can vary over a wide range, although it is typically on the order of 10% to 20%.[18] Another concern is that contaminants, such as pesticides and heavy metals, have also been identified in some lecithin preparations.[18] Clinicians would be well-advised, therefore, to restrict the medicinal use of lecithin at this time to carefully designed protocols involving systematic collection of data, informed consent, defined lecithin preparations, and monitoring of plasma choline concentrations.[19]

REFERENCES

1. Baldessarini RJ, Tarsy D: Tardive dyskinesia, in Lipton MA, DiMascio A, Killam KF (eds): *Psychopharmacology: A Generation of Progress.* New York, Raven Press, 1978, pp 993–1004.
2. Jeste DV, Wyatt RJ: In search of treatments for tardive dyskinesia: Review of the literature. *Schizo Bull* 5:251–293, 1979.
3. Cohen EL, Wurtman RJ: Brain acetylcholine: Control by dietary choline. *Science* 191:561–562, 1976.
4. Haubrich DR, Wang PFL, Clody DE, et al: Increase in brain acetylcholine induced by choline or deanol. *Life Sci* 17:975–980, 1975.
5. Davis KL, Berger PA, Hollister LE: Choline for tardive dyskinesia (letter to editor). *N Engl J Med* 293:152, 1975.
6. Davis KL, Berger PA, Hollister LE: Clinical and preclinical experience with choline chloride in Huntington's disease and tardive dyskinesia: Unanswered questions, in Barbeau A, Growdon JH, Wurtman RJ (eds): *Nutrition and the Brain. Volume 5: Choline and Lecithin in Brain Diseases.* New York, Raven Press, 1979, pp 305–316.
7. Tamminga CA, Smith RC, Ericksen SE, et al: Cholinergic influences in tardive dyskinesia. *Am J Psychiatry* 134:769–774, 1977.
8. Growdon, JH, Hirsch MJ, Wurtman RJ, et al: Oral choline administration to patients with tardive dyskinesia. *N Engl J Med* 297:524–527, 1977.
9. Wurtman JJ: Sources of choline and lecithin in the diet, in Barbeau A, Growdon JH, Wurtman RJ (eds): *Nutrition and the Brain. Volume 5: Choline and Lecithin in Brain Diseases.* New York, Raven Press, 1979, pp 73–82.
10. Hirsch MJ, Wurtman RJ: Lecithin consumption increases acetylcholine concentrations in rat brain and adrenal medulla. *Science* 202:223–225, 1978.
11. Wurtman RJ, Hirsch MJ, Growdon JH: Lecithin consumption raises serum-free-choline levels. *Lancet* 2:68–69, 1977.

12. Gelenberg AJ, Wojcik JD, Growdon JH: Lecithin for the treatment of tardive dyskinesia, in Barbeau A, Growdon JH, Wurtman RJ (eds): *Nutrition and the Brain. Volume 5: Choline and Lecithin in Brain Disorders.* New York, Raven Press, 1979, pp 417–424.

13. Barbeau A: Lecithin in movement disorders, in Barbeau A, Growdon JH, Wurtman RJ (eds): *Nutrition and the Brain. Volume 5: Choline and Lecithin in Brain Disorders.* New York, Raven Press, 1979, pp 263–272.

14. Jackson IV, Nuttall EA, Ibe IO, et al: Treatment of tardive dyskinesia with lecithin. *Am J Psychiatry* 136:1458–1460, 1979.

15. Branchey MH, Branchey LB, Bark NM, Richardson MA: Lecithin in the treatment of tardive dyskinesia. *Commun Psychopharmacol* 3:303–307, 1979.

16. Growdon JH: Neurotransmitter precursors in the diet: Their use in the treatment of brain diseases, in Wurtman RJ, Wurtman JJ (eds): *Nutrition and the Brain. Volume 3: Disorders of Eating and Nutrients in Treatment of Brain Diseases.* New York, Raven Press, 1979, pp 117–182.

17. Gelenberg AJ: Nutrition in psychiatry, editorial. *J Clin Psychiatry* 41:328, 1980.

18. Hanin I: Commercially available 'lecithin:' Proposed guidelines for nomenclature and methodology, in Barbeau A, Growdon JH, Wurtman RJ (eds): *Nutrition and the Brain. Volume 5: Choline and Lecithin in Brain Disorders.* New York, Raven Press, 1979, pp 443–446.

19. Gelenberg AJ: Lecithin for tardive dyskinesia. *MGH Biol Ther Psychiatry Newsl* 2:47, 1979.

14

Prediction and Prevention of Tardive Dyskinesia

Panel Discussion

Joseph DeVeaugh-Geiss
James M. Smith
Richard L. Borison
Donald M. Pirodsky
Eric D. Caine
Alan J. Gelenberg
Guy Chouinard

Basically, our concern is prevention, although any information that will enable the prediction of the development of tardive dyskinesia in a patient will also be clinically useful. The reason prevention becomes so important is that there are no *good* treatments for patients who develop tardive dyskinesia. If it can be prevented, our patients will be better off.

Doctor Borison reported in his study that he found prochlorperazine (Compazine) and haloperidol (Haldol) to have higher affinity for striatal dopamine receptors in relationship to limbic affinity, whereas thioridazine (Mellaril) and clozapine had apparently higher affinity for the limbic receptors (see Chapter 11). I would like to add to this some clinical findings consistent with his data. Suzanne Miller and I have recently examined 250 chronically institutionalized patients, and among these, 44 patients have taken only one neuroleptic (see Figure 14-1). Because of the variety of drugs represented in this sample, the number of patients in many of the groups is too small for adequate statistical analysis. It is very clear, however, when referring to the AIMS scores (see Appendix II),

162

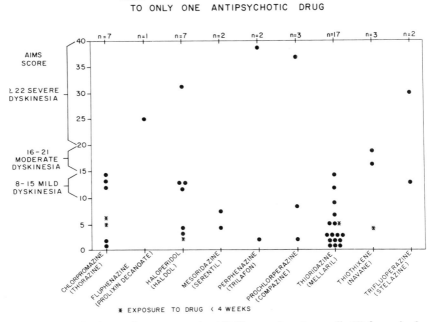

AIMS RATINGS OF 44 PATIENTS EXPOSED
TO ONLY ONE ANTIPSYCHOTIC DRUG

Figure 14-1 Each • or * represents the AIMS score (see Appendix II) for a single patient. Mild dyskinesia (AIMS = 8–15) scores had at least one item rated as mild, and no items rated as moderate or severe. Moderate dyskinesia (AIMS = 16–21) scores had at least one item rated as moderate and no items rated as severe. Severe dyskinesia (AIMS = 22–40) had at least one item rated as severe.

which can range from 0 to 42, that the patients chronically maintained on thioridazine cluster around the low AIMS scores, while the patients with the highest scores, in the 30s and high 20s, were taking the high potency neuroleptics. Three of the drugs represented in this sample (chlorpromazine, thioridazine, and haloperidol) were taken by enough patients to permit statistical analysis with the Mann-Whitney U test. From this study, it can be concluded that the likelihood of a higher score on the AIMS scale is greater with haloperidol (p = .02) and with chlorpromazine (p = .05) than with thioridazine. The sample sizes were insufficient to permit comparison of the haloperidol and chlorpromazine groups with each other. While we must keep in mind the limitations of findings derived from retrospective studies such as this one, we find these data interesting and consistent with Doctor Borison's findings. In addition, the correlation of higher dyskinesia scores with the use of the more potent neuroleptics also corresponds to the incidence of acute, parkinsonian side effects seen with these drugs, which leads to my comments about prediction of tardive dyskinesia.

Please keep in mind that the first step in the pathogenesis of tardive dyskinesia is blockade of striatal dopamine (DA) receptors (see Chapter 1). According to current hypotheses, a person cannot develop tardive dyskinesia without this; so if a drug can block striatal DA receptors, and the drug is good at blocking these receptors, it is likely to predispose to dyskinesia. The other thing that corresponds clinically with blockade of dopamine receptors in the striatum is extrapyramidal side effects (EPS) of the parkinsonian type. In my opinion, persistent EPS are a predisposing factor for tardive dyskinesia. I do not believe that this is true for EPS that appear and remit spontaneously, but only for persistent EPS.

I have made a clinical observation, which seems somewhat unusual, insofar as it does not correspond to anything learned previously in my training, but I found something quite like it in the early literature on neuroleptics. I call it the marching syndrome. A young man who had very subtle oral facial dyskinesia, which followed a course of acute hypokinetic extrapyramidal side effects — parkinsonism with tremor — on a maintenance dose of neuroleptic, progressed to a hyperkinetic rigidity; that is, he was moving more rapidly, accompanied by akathisia, which then progressed to a more choreiform and oral facial movement disorder. In the early literature, a report by Gerald Sarwer-Foner from 1960 describes akathisia: "The patients feel they must keep moving and pacing, they have restless feet." Interesting in this report, though, is the description of this restlessness. "Patients describe the feeling of being driven with an increased feeling of tension, a feeling of pulling or drawing in the extremities, chiefly in the legs."[1] And he further describes that people pace back and forth, etc. Some other reports in the early literature also seem to describe something that I have seen: long-lasting hyperkinesias described by Delay and Deniker in 1968. "Long-lasting hyperkinesias may consist of akathisia and tasikinesia (tendency to continue moving), with a compulsion to walk or to carry out a maneuver like *soldiers marking time.*"[2] Another relevant report from 1961 by Denham and Carrick characterizes side effects of neuroleptics. They describe the akinetic state, the akineto-hypertonic state, and the hyperkineto-hypertonic state, which is what I am describing, and this is differentiated from the others by the presence of motor restlessness. "The patient must walk about constantly and is not satisfied with standing still . . . he feels that something is pushing him, that he has to constantly move . . . movements of the feet *resembling a dilatory form of marking time* occurred in all the patients who displayed akathisia."[3] So, they are differentiating the marching movements from the akathisia. While following a group of five people longitudinally who have shown this condition, I observed that they do not all have akathisia. They are marching around, but not necessarily because they feel that they have to keep moving; some have akathisia, and some do not. All of these patients have shown a very clear progression of symptoms from an acute extrapyramidal parkinsonian reaction, which is hypokinetic with shuffling gait, to a more hyperkinetic, still rigid, marching kind of a movement, and progression from that to choreoathetosis and orofacial dyskinesia.

CASE REPORTS

1. The first example of this marching syndrome occurred in a 31-year-old man who was being treated with chlorpromazine 500 mg daily and benztropine 4 mg daily. During the third week of this therapy he developed parkinsonian side effects, which consisted of tremor, rigidity, shuffling gait, and pronounced bradykinesia. During the fourth week, this shifted from a hypokinetic rigidity to a hyperkinetic rigidity, while the tremor persisted. He had definite muscular rigidity with a stiff posture and gait, but rather than shuffling his gait was characterized by "marching" in which he raised his feet and knees high into the air as he walked. He also displayed this hyperkinesia while standing still, and he truly gave the appearance of a soldier "marking time." During the fifth week, he developed mild puckering of the lips and tongue protrusions. At this point, the benztropine was discontinued, and within 24 hours, the syndrome, including the orofacial component, worsened considerably. Chlorpromazine was discontinued and the rigidity, gait disturbance, and orofacial dyskinesia completely disappeared within 72 hours. Thus, although an orofacial dyskinesia was present, pharmacologically this behaved like an acute parkinsonian side effect; ie, it worsened when the anticholinergic drug was discontinued, and improved when the neuroleptic was discontinued. (See Chapter 1 for pharmacology of extrapyramidal movement disorders, and also Chapter 8, *Differential Diagnosis.*)

2. A 30-year-old man who was receiving trifluoperazine 30 mg daily developed a typical parkinsonian reaction that was treated with benztropine 4 mg daily during the first three weeks of therapy. This drug regimen was maintained, and a very similar shift from hypokinetic to hyperkinetic rigidity developed. The "marching syndrome" in this man was allowed to persist for several weeks until blepharospasm, grimacing, lingual dyskinesia, and limb chorea were noticed. At this time the drugs were discontinued, and a frank buccal-lingual-facial dyskinesia with chorea of all four extremities emerged. Although these involuntary movements improved somewhat while the patient was off medications, a residual dyskinesia of moderate degree has persisted for nearly two years.

3. A 62-year-old man was referred with signs of muscular rigidity and restless legs. On examination he showed rigidity, parkinsonian posture with decreased arm swing, and abnormal gait characterized by high elevation of the knees while standing still and while walking. He clearly appeared to be marching in place. There was also mild grimacing observable in the facial musculature but no significant signs of tardive dyskinesia, all of this occurring while he received a maintenance dose of neuroleptic. In an effort to characterize this phenomenon pharmacologically, he was given benztropine 4 mg daily with no change in neuroleptic dosage, and his parkinsonian symptoms diminished: his gait improved, there was some arm swing as he walked, the rigidity abated, and the marching was substantially reduced. His orofacial movements, however, worsened, so that the grimacing was more pronounced. He appeared to exhibit the classical response to anticholinergic challenge, ie, improvement in parkinsonism and worsening of dyskinesia. When neuroleptics were withdrawn, the parkinsonism disappeared completely and a full orofacial dyskinesia with abnormal buccal, lingual, and masticatory movements, as well as blepharospasm appeared. After approximately six weeks, the dyskinesia began to improve and subsequently disappeared completely. The history provided by the referring physician documented clearly that the patient had developed a typical parkinsonian extrapyramidal reaction with shuffling gait, which had then progressed to the marching gait after about eight weeks on neuroleptics.

4. A 58-year-old man developed tardive dyskinesia after many years of neuroleptic therapy and was referred for withdrawal from neuroleptics. He was observed to also have the marching gait and muscular rigidity. History revealed that he had this gait disturbance for at least six months, and that his neuroleptic dosage had been the same during that period of time. Withdrawal from neuroleptic resulted in improvement in the gait disturbance and loss of rigidity, accompanied by marked increase in orofacial dyskinesia, with choreiform involuntary movements of the lower extremities. Over the next six months, there was a gradual improvement of the dyskinesia, but it has persisted for more than one year. This patient also had a well-documented parkinsonian reaction with shuffling gait prior to the onset of the marching gait. Although appearing to have restless legs, he did not have a subjective sense of restlessness; that is, he had no akathisia.

5. A 35-year-old man with parkinsonian extrapyramidal side effects, including shuffling gait and rigidity while taking haloperidol 20 mg daily for four weeks, gradually developed the rigid, marching syndrome described with no signs of orofacial dyskinesia, accompanied by akathisia. When the neuroleptic was discontinued during the sixth week of therapy, the akathisia remitted as well as the parkinsonian symptoms,

and he developed abnormal movements of the tongue and jaw, which disappeared within three weeks.

It appears from these cases that the extrapyramidal side effects of neuroleptic drugs may progress from a hypokinetic to a hyperkinetic state and that the two may coexist, suggesting that drug-induced parkinsonism and tardive dyskinesia may represent the extremes of a continuum or spectrum of extrapyramidal movement disorders. It has been postulated that there are two distinct types of dopaminergic neurons, each one responsible for either the parkinsonian or dyskinetic side effects. What is striking, and probably most important, about these cases, is that tardive dyskinesia may be covertly present while parkinsonian rigidity persists (and perhaps masks the dyskinesia), and that akathisia may occur independently of the hyperactivity and motor restlessness seen during this stage.

Clinical experience informs us that not all patients with parkinsonian extrapyramidal reactions show signs of dyskinesia when neuroleptics are discontinued, yet all of my patients with the marching syndrome manifested dyskinesia. Although documentation of this progression from hypokinetic rigidity to tardive dyskinesia in a large number of patients would be necessary before firm conclusions could be drawn, I would propose that patients who develop the hyperkinetic rigidity, or marching syndrome, described here may already have covert dyskinesia, and should be considered as a population at high risk for tardive dyskinesia. Furthermore, I am suggesting that this may be one of the early signs of incipient dyskinesia, and that drug withdrawal at this point may precipitate a dyskinesia that is more likely to be reversible than would be the case if the patient remained on the neuroleptic drug until overt signs of dyskinesia were present.

Joseph DeVeaugh-Geiss

REFERENCES

1. Sarwer-Foner GJ: Recognition and management of drug-induced extrapyramidal reactions and "paradoxical" behavioural reactions in psychiatry. *Can Med Assoc J* 83:312–318, 1960.

2. Delay J, Deniker P: Drug-induced extrapyramidal syndromes, in Vinken PJ, Bruyn GW (eds): *Diseases of the Basal Ganglia (Handbook of Clinical Neurology, vol 6.* Amsterdam, North Holland Publishing Corp, 1968, pp 248–266.

3. Denham J, Carrick DJEL: Therapeutic value of thioproperazine and the importance of the associated neurological disturbances. *J Ment Science* 107:326–345, 1961.

*   *   *   *

There are a few trends as well as some other things related to tardive dyskinesia which have emerged from our review of the literature. The first is that most people are fairly well in agreement that dyskinesia is frequently reversible in younger patients, especially when it is detected early. Based on a study by Jeste and associates, which was published in the May 1979, *Archives of General Psychiatry,* it appears that even among older patients – chronic patients, average age 60 years, average length of hospitalization 20 years – there is considerable remission upon drug withdrawal. They reported a 57% remission rate within the first three months of discontinuation of neuroleptics. People have quoted that study to support the opinion that tardive dyskinesia is probably reversible even in these older, chronically hospitalized patients. Our own follow-up data of 139 patients indicates that the group taken off neuroleptics for an average of a year and a half are significantly worse off the neuroleptics than they were three years ago when they were on the neuroleptics. Not all of them had been off drug for three years but they have had a fairly long time off neuroleptics. If the syndrome is going to disappear in the first three months, as Jeste's report suggests, then many of these patients should have been much better by the time we re-rated them three years later. So, many chronic patients will not have reversible dyskinesia.

A related problem is what to do for chronic patients manifesting tardive dyskinesia. Our results indicate that if neuroleptics are discontinued, then many patients are not going to get better. That would seem to imply that switching to another neuroleptic probably would not be very helpful either. It should also be mentioned that the APA task force studying late-appearing neurological disorders, chaired by Doctor Ross Baldessarini, has summarized the results of ten studies of remission following the withdrawal of neuroleptics and found an average percent remission somewhere in the low twenties. So there again the results are not very encouraging in terms of reversibility.

The second trend, again of note on the basis of the literature review, is that there is a fair amount of evidence indicating that, in a rather sizable number of patients, the original development of tardive dyskinesia occurs within the first three to five years of treatment. It is important, therefore, to be very alert during the early stages of neuroleptic treatment and not to assume that tardive dyskinesia only occurs after patients have received treatment for many years. In contrast, we may be able to get very early indications that some patients are not going to respond to treatment, and I would be more cautious in those patients who have the relatively early onset, insidious development of their psychotic disorder. Some of the literature suggests that these patients may be more susceptible to developing tardive dyskinesia.

One last fact, although not directly related to tardive dyskinesia, but certainly indirectly, is that there is a growing realization that patients can be maintained on much lower doses of neuroleptics than ever thought possible previously. The low dose fluphenazine (Prolixin) studies indicate that rather clearly. In addition, some recent data on neuroleptic blood levels and therapeutic response by Van Putten and others, have suggested that some patients seem to do quite well even with blood levels that would normally be considered subtherapeutic.

James M. Smith

*   *   *   *

We have heard about a number of different movement disorders during this symposium, and have highlighted the fact that it is sometimes very difficult to make a proper diagnosis. Just because a patient has a particular body part that is shaking does not necessarily mean that the patient has tardive dyskinesia, Tourette's syndrome or another movement disorder. It is important to recognize the difference between a tic, as in Tourette's, and a choreiform movement disorder; a tic is a quick movement and a choreiform movement is slower. There are different gradations and sometimes it is very difficult to distinguish one from another. For example, the rabbit syndrome, which is a tremor of the upper lip — the patient looks somewhat like a rabbit — resembles parkinsonian tremor and tardive dyskinesia. Usually, one thinks that any facial-lingual-buccal involvement must be tardive dyskinesia, but the rabbit syndrome frequently responds to anticholinergic drugs, ie, benztropine mesylate (Cogentin), and this is probably a parkinsonian type of side effect. One has to be very careful in the evaluation and treatment of these movement disorders because an anticholinergic drug that might be useful in treating parkinsonian side effects should not be used in a patient with dyskinesia. Also, in terms of the pharmacology, the dopamine-acetyl choline balance hypothesis and the notion of a preponderance of dopamine relative to acetyl choline in tardive dyskinesia may also be inadequate (see Chapters 1 and 8). Some pharmacological studies suggest that there are patients for whom that actually seems to be reversed. Studies by Daniel Casey, giving physostigmine and anticholinergic challenges to patients, indicate that some patients respond in a manner opposite to that expected, ie, worsening with cholinergic treatment and improving with anticholinergic treatment. Therefore, one should not have a monolithic point of view in terms of recognizing and treating movement disorders. It is important to look carefully at the patient to see what is happening.

In regard to Doctor Smith's comments: the retrospective studies are our best sources of information, but there are problems with these studies and probably few people besides Doctor Smith realize the Herculean task it is to do such studies. Nevertheless, prospective studies would be a better approach because cause and effect relationships with retrospective studies are difficult to assess. Considering that all of the antipsychotic drugs, some a little more than others, are very potent in masking dyskinesias, it becomes difficult to retrospectively determine when a person first developed dyskinesia if he received many different drugs over a period of years. Did it develop while he took chlorpromazine (Thorazine) in 1964, or when he took haloperidol (Haldol) in 1975, or when he took thiothixene (Navane) in 1980? This makes it very difficult to pinpoint, in retrospective studies, whether certain drugs have a greater likelihood of producing tardive dyskinesia than other drugs because there are so few studies where one patient has been followed while taking only one antipsychotic drug.

It is important to remember, as Doctor Smith pointed out, that patients can develop tardive dyskinesia much earlier than we previously thought. To my knowledge the earliest occurring tardive dyskinesia reported is after four months. I saw a patient who, after seven months on fluphenazine (Prolixin), developed a full blown tardive dyskinesia which has proven to be persistent. Tardive dyskinesia can occur early in treatment but, as long as the patient continues to take an antipsychotic drug, it can remain a covert dyskinesia — it can be masked by the drug. Remember that there are withdrawal dyskinesias, covert dyskinesias, and tardive dyskinesias — the purely reversible to perhaps the irreversible — and they might be thought of as existing on a spectrum. With early detection many studies have shown that the syndrome is reversible. As long as it is covert, or masked by the antipsychotic drug, it will be difficult to detect. There have been a few prospective studies that have been done and Doctor DeVeaugh-Geiss's is an important one.

At the International Phenothiazine Symposium in Zurich, Switzerland, in September, 1979, Axelson and other Scandinavian investigators reported that among a group of patients receiving only thioridazine (Mellaril) over a ten-year period none developed tardive dyskinesia. This does not mean that thioridazine produces no tardive dyskinesia. Any antipsychotic drug has the potential for producing tardive dyskinesia, but certainly with more prospective studies, we might be able to better identify those drugs which may have a lower likelihood of producing tardive dyskinesia. And there are several antipsychotic drugs available in Europe that appear to have low potential for producing tardive dyskinesia. Prochlorperazine (Compazine) was mentioned earlier (see Chapter 11). I do not use prochlorperazine clinically, even as an anti-emetic, and it is not used as an antipsychotic drug. An interesting thing about prochlorperazine is that it demonstrates a site specificity in the brain. It is very potent as an antiemetic and in producing extrapyramidal side effects, but relatively weak as an antipsychotic drug. Clozapine is ex-actly the opposite, ie, it is a good antipsychotic drug, but does not pro-duce extrapyramidal side effects and has virtually no antiemetic proper-ties. Between clozapine and prochlorperazine we have a whole range of drugs with varying degrees of these major effects and side effects. Thioridazine is more like clozapine, while some other antipsychotic drugs tend to be more like prochlorperazine, and many of the newer European drugs tend to be more like clozapine (see also Chapter 11).

Another important consideration in choosing antipsychotic drugs for patients is the risk/benefit ratio (see Chapter 15). It is very important from a medical/legal point of view to document that one went through this decision-making process. In the final analysis, the courts are prob-ably going to be more interested in knowing that one has clinically evaluated risks *vs* benefits rather than other supplementary things, such as informed consent. A good clinician working in the patient's best in-terest is aware of the pitfalls in giving antipsychotic drugs, and with ade-quate documentation of this awareness it will be difficult for anyone to find fault with what the physician has done.

One question raised had to do with inheriting a patient who had been previously treated by others. If one then reduces the medication and uncovers covert dyskinesia, and the patient then decides to sue, who will be stuck with the lawsuit? Any physician who has treated a patient can be named in a lawsuit, but the doctor's liability might be minimal if he can demonstrate that he was doing his job as a physician and was looking for these things. As more lawsuits are apparent, we will be better able to establish guidelines in terms of legal aspects of tardive dyskinesia (see Chapter 15). But again, as long as the physician is not negligent, is aware of this potential problem, is looking for it, and is documenting this in the medical record, then his liability is probably going to be very minimal.

Richard L. Borison

*   *   *   *

I have a few brief comments — one is philosophical in nature and the other is practical. The best way to deal with tardive dyskinesia right now is primary prevention. This means using less medication or perhaps not using it at all. There have been more lawsuits initiated as a result of people having this syndrome, which is obviously going to affect the way physicians prescribe medications. There are going to be a lot of people who may not want to use these medications at all, even when they are indicated. One has to consider how that will change the practice of psychiatry. Over the past quarter of a century that antipsychotics have been available, a striking shift in the balance of in-patient and out-patient psychiatric populations has been seen. One can only speculate what the future holds. Are we going to see a reversal of this trend? The answer is not yet known, but the practice of psychiatry is going to be affected in some ways.

As a consultation/liaison psychiatrist, I am also interested in drug prescription by other medical specialists. Psychiatrists are becoming more aware of tardive dyskinesia, but is this same increasing awareness shared by other medical specialists? Frankly, when I go around on the wards, I am amazed at how frequently psychotropic drugs are casually prescribed. It is often a knee-jerk reaction when a resident hears from the nurse, "Doctor, this patient is having trouble sleeping at night," and for flurazepam (Dalmane) to be ordered in the chart. One thing you may not be aware of is that 70% of all psychotropics are prescribed by non-psychiatrists. Granted, that includes a lot of chlordiazepoxide (Librium) and diazepam (Valium), but it also includes antipsychotics and tricyclics. Doctor Borison's comments are particularly pertinent in this regard. I do not know many psychiatrists who are prescribing prochlorperazine (Compazine), but I do know a lot of other physicians in the community who are. Are they aware of the risk of tardive dyskinesia? There is a need, not only for psychiatrists, but for other medical specialists also, to better understand this syndrome. Part of our role should be educating our colleagues about psychotropic drugs.

Donald M. Pirodsky

*   *   *   *

I would like to offer some specific examples of ways to reduce medication. A current problem is rapid neuroleptization. What we effectively treat with rapid neuroleptization is a combative, argumentative, negative, hostile, threatening, and violent patient who frightens us and others. When we rapidly neurolepticize such a patient he will go to sleep. Now that may be well and good and, indeed, very helpful and effective as management, but there is more than one way to deal with that situation. Usually, I try to treat people who present in that state of mind with the dose of neuroleptic drug that I want to maintain. For example, I may start someone on 20 to 40 mg of haloperidol (Haldol), which is not going to put them to sleep. There are other ways to make people go to sleep, or at least to make people drowsy and more tranquil. In this connection, I would mention a study in the *American Journal of Psychiatry* published in August of 1979 comparing intravenous diazepam (Valium) with intravenous haloperidol which showed that, within 24 hours, diazepam had as substantial an "antipsychotic" effect as did haloperidol. I do not think that diazepam is an antipsychotic drug, but the items often rated and the things thought of as related to "psychosis" on these rating scales really are not psychotic items, but are agitation. Recall the early psychopharmacology drug trials where the difference between active antipsychotic drug and placebo was not seen in week one or week two, but began appearing in weeks three, four, five and six. As with antidepressant drugs, the therapeutic effects of neuroleptic drugs are not seen overnight, but more often they are seen after the drug has been administered over a period of weeks. There appears to be a need for some sort of adjustment to the medication, and the psychiatrists in the 1960s were probably aware of this when they established certain kinds of drug treatment regimens.

A second type of problem frequently confronted is a psychopharmacology consult where there is no question about whether the patient received enough medication or was tried on one or another kind of drug. Indeed, these patients have been treated very "effectively" as far as the usual steps are concerned and they have not improved. In this situation, there is an indication for stopping medication and reassessing the patient, and certainly *not* an indication for continuing high dose drug treatment. If one considers the target symptoms that one is attempting to treat, such as thought disorder, hallucinations, and delusions, and if these do not respond to "effective" treatment, then one must reconsider the diagnosis and consider whether or not the patient could be expected to respond to treatment with medication. Such items as poor judgment, constricted affect, and problems with memory or orientation are notoriously bad responders to antipsychotic drugs in any event, and certainly one has to wonder whether these symptoms are worthy of treatment, because if a good response cannot be expected and the patient might get a tardive dyskinesia, then the risk/benefit ratio changes (see Chapter 15). For young, psychotic people who have not responded to antipsychotic drugs after three to five months I frequently recommend that they consider a course of ECT, and I take them off medication. This opinion is based primarily on the work of Phillip May who suggested that the longer a patient remains psychotic the worse the prognosis will be. So, if a psychotic patient has had effective dopamine receptor blockade by a number of different kinds of neuroleptic drugs, then perhaps another approach to treatment is indicated.

There are several areas in which we should think most carefully about what we are doing. We want to use the lowest effective dose of medication and there may be several ways to achieve this. Certainly, there are many people in outpatient clinics who are on maintenance neuroleptics and are not much better for the medicine they receive. These people need careful and *gradual* dose reduction; because the risk of relapse is greater if dose reduction is done quickly. Then, a careful evaluation of how the patient is doing, along with social support during and after the change in medication, will help to reduce the risk of relapse.

An interesting thing that emerges from these considerations is almost a circular problem. One generally thinks in terms of seeing chronic patients, attempting to lower their dose, and looking for signs of tardive dyskinesia. So a patient who has been taking trifluoperazine (Stelazine) 10 mg daily for the past 10 or 20 years, has a dose reduction for two weeks, suddenly develops abnormal involuntary movements, and then has emergent psychotic symptoms. At this point one realizes that this situation might have been easier to understand three years ago, before Doctor Chouinard brought up the idea of tardive psychosis (see Chapter 9). Three years ago, one might have concluded that the patient was still psychotic and continued to need antipsychotic medication. But now, considering that the emergent psychotic symptoms could represent a tardive psychosis, one does not know whether to take the patient off the medication, to resume it, to slowly decrease the dose, or to do something else, because on the one hand there is evidence of abnormal involuntary movements, and on the other hand the patient may have a tardive psychosis. Things are becoming both clear and cloudy at the same time.

One thing that I routinely attempt is to avoid abruptly stopping medication in favor of systematically tapering the dose. For the first psychotic episode, I will begin to slowly reduce medication dosage after four to five months, and usually plan to discontinue all medications over a period of two to three months. For some chronic patients this may amount to only reducing their fluphenazine dose by spacing the injections a little bit further apart. This approach may help answer the question of whether a tardive psychosis may be accompanying the abnormal involuntary movements, because gradual dose reduction may result in breakthrough of movement disorder without the mental status aberrations frequently seen when neuroleptic drugs are abruptly discontinued. There is a great deal of uncertainty in the management of patients withdrawn from neuroleptic drugs. We may end up putting people back on medicine for mental status problems that emerged when drugs were reduced or discontinued, but which would not have occurred if their medication dosage had been gradually discontinued.

We need to acknowledge that there are some people who do not respond to drug treatments, or to any other approaches that are currently available, and that the treatment alternatives for these people are very limited. We must recognize that certain schizophrenic syndromes are persistent and progressive and that medications are not the right thing for these patients, possibly because they have a different pathogenesis compared with the other schizophrenic syndromes that respond very nicely and very rapidly to drug treatment. There is a spectrum of disease processes that we face and some of these people probably will remain institutionalized (see Chapter 15). I would hope that the institution would not necessarily have to be large, with high walls and chainlink fences, but this is a societal decision. Similarly, patients having disabling tardive dyskinesia will not help the situation, and it is important to attempt to separate out the different issues.

Eric D. Caine

*   *   *   *

Our fondest hope would be to find non-neuroleptic antipsychotic drugs; that is to say, drugs that could combat the symptoms of psychosis without producing neurologic effects. Clozapine, a dibenzoxazepine derivative, appeared to fill this bill. Some preclinical data suggested that clozapine might have blocked dopamine receptors selectively in mesolimbic and mesocortical networks (the presumed locus of antipsychotic efficacy), while being a relatively weak dopamine blocker in the nigrostriatal and tuberoinfundibular pathways (which control extrapyramidal movements and prolactin secretion, respectively). Thus, while effectively alleviating hallucinations, delusions, and disorganized thinking, clozapine produced few or no extrapyramidal effects, probably did not cause tardive dyskinesia, and had little prolactin-elevating potential. Unfortunately, clozapine was probably associated with a higher incidence of agranulocytosis than other antipsychotic agents, which resulted in its withdrawal from clinical investigation in the United States and from a large market in many other countries. Despite its relatively brief sojourn with us, however, clozapine taught us that the search for non-neuroleptic antipsychotic drugs, which presumably will free us from the dilemma of tardive dyskinesia, is not without hope (see also Chapters 8 and 11).

For the time being, our best prospects lie in conservative use of the drugs currently available. I doubt that any one of the antipsychotic drugs we now prescribe is safer or that any is more deleterious regarding liability of producing tardive dyskinesia. While thioridazine (Mellaril), for example, is associated with a lower incidence of acute extrapyramidal effects, there is no evidence of a lower incidence of tardive dyskinesia in association with the use of this drug than with other drugs. Moreover, data from Clow et al in England suggests that chronic administration of thioridazine, much like chronic administration of high-potency phenothiazines, can lead to supersensitivity at the striatal dopamine receptor, which is thought to underlie tardive dyskinesia.

To reiterate, the best approach to dealing with tardive dyskinesia is conservative use of neuroleptic agents. Thus, their prescription to alleviate problems in living, mild cases of anxiety, and nonpsychotic depression should be discouraged, especially if nonbiological therapy or less toxic drugs may be considered (see Chapter 6).

When antipsychotic agents are clearly indicated, the best advice is to use the lowest effective dose for the shortest period of time. This means that when a patient is being treated chronically, periodic reassessment of antipsychotic drug dose is in order. Many chronic schizophrenic patients can be maintained on relatively low dosages of these drugs, and probably 20% to 35% of them will remain symptom free for a year or more with no medication.

In addition, when patients are maintained chronically on these agents, they should be examined once or twice a year for early signs of abnormal, involuntary movements. If these movements are observed, serious consideration should be given to tapering and discontinuing the antipsychotic drug. For medical-legal purposes, the chart should note that the dose was periodically reassessed, the patient had been screened for abnormal movements, and that these matters had been discussed with the patient and family.

Clearly, better antipsychotic drugs are needed. Our present armamentarium carries the unfortunate risk of tardive dyskinesia. Moreover, the drugs we now have leave untouched the so-called negative symptoms of schizophrenia, such as flattened affect, social isolation, and withdrawal. Nevertheless, phenothiazines and related compounds have allowed many chronic schizophrenics to reside outside of hospitals, free from institutional restrictions, and liberated from previously debilitating psychotic symptoms. Hence, until we have a new generation of more effective and less toxic antipsychotic drugs, our present drugs should be used to the best advantage of patients suffering from the ravages of psychotic illnesses. But, the drugs must be used wisely and conservatively if the cure is not to be worse then the disease.

Alan J. Gelenberg

*   *   *   *

There are several recommendations that can be made to prevent the development of tardive dyskinesia. The first, as discussed by Doctor

Caine, is the tapering of neuroleptic medication. It is in this regard that the concept of tardive psychosis is most important, since recognizing the syndrome will prevent patients from receiving escalating doses of medication. Thus, even if the patient is a little paranoid at the end of the injection period or when a dose of medication is missed, we find it beneficial to decrease the medication every six months or so to achieve the minimum therapeutic dosage. This is further facilitated by the use of high potency neuroleptics, which have fewer side effects upon withdrawal than do the low potency neuroleptics.

Secondly, one should try to adjust the dosage regimen so that the tardive dyskinesia can be uncovered. If a patient is taking neuroleptics four times a day, it is nearly impossible to see tardive dyskinesia because of the covering effect of the medication. Thus, after a patient has been treated for a number of weeks we try to decrease the medication to once a day or, if possible, every second day. In this way, any tardive dyskinesia will be more obvious and prevention can be begun immediately. The dose regimen appears to be the main factor explaining the discrepancy between early surveys of tardive dyskinesia and the more recent ones (see Chapters 3 and 4). Early surveys were carried out in populations taking neuroleptics four times a day. It is only recently that this factor has been recognized and patients on a once-a-day regimen or on depot neuroleptics every two to three weeks have been surveyed.

Third, another way to prevent tardive dyskinesia is to carefully examine patients at the time the blood level of neuroleptics is at its lowest. For patients on IM medication, this is at the end of the injection interval; for those on oral medication, it is necessary to question the patient closely on the effects of a missed dose. A thorough examination can often detect the initial signs of tardive dyskinesia.

The fourth method recommended is the use of anticholinergic drugs, which is presently a controversial issue. It has been argued by Doctor Tanner and associates that the long-term use of anticholinergic drugs exacerbates tardive dyskinesia.[1] The subject needs further investigation and at this time no long-term controlled study has, to our knowledge, shown that the use of anticholinergic drugs may be harmful. In any event, it was found that, in a study of 260 schizophrenic patients chronically treated with neuroleptic drugs, the use of anticholinergic drugs was not a factor related to the development of tardive dyskinesia.[2] Also, exacerbation of tardive dyskinesia by temporary administration of an anticholinergic drug could be reversed to previous baseline severity by discontinuing the drug.[3] Christensen and Nielsen[4] have demonstrated that the administration of anticholinergic drugs in mice during the phase of dopaminergic supersensitivity development induced by neuroleptics had no influence on the development of that supersensitivity.

Hogarty found that 98% of his patients needed antiparkinsonian drugs at one time or another during his study.[5] Also, Jellinek and associates, at the 1980 American Psychiatric Association meeting presented results showing that 60% of his patients had emergence of parkinsonian symptoms on withdrawal of medication.[6] Both of these studies are in agreement with our own findings, that most patients require the use of anticholinergic drugs at one time or another when they are being treated with high potency neuroleptics. From our study on long-acting depot neuroleptics, it is estimated that 70% to 80% of patients needed an antiparkinsonian drug during long-term maintenance treatment.[7]

Our policy for the control of tardive dyskinesia is always to avoid anything that covers up the syndrome, which hypokinetic parkinsonism definitely does. Thus, the use of antiparkinsonian drugs, on the short-term at least, is a way to try to uncover, and therefore deal with, tardive dyskinesia.

In summary, the best prevention for tardive dyskinesia is achieved by the administration of the lowest therapeutic dose of neuroleptics. This can be most readily achieved by the recognition of supersensitivity psychosis and by the use of high-potency neuroleptics, which have fewer withdrawal effects facilitating dose reduction. In addition, it is important to avoid covering up tardive dyskinesia as this leads to more severe forms of the disorder. This is achieved by: 1) the use of once-a-day regimens for oral medication, or bimonthly or monthly injections for patients on injectable neuroleptics, 2) by preventing parkinsonism, which tends to mask tardive dyskinesia, and 3) by the coadministration of an anticholinergic, antiparkinsonian agent, which tends to uncover tardive dyskinesia.

Guy Chouinard

REFERENCES

1. Tanner C, Goetz CG, Weiner WJ: Anticholinergics and tardive dyskinesia. Letters to the Editor, *Am J Psychiatry* 137:1470, 1980.

2. Chouinard G, Annable L, Ross-Chouinard A, et al: Factors related to tardive dyskinesia. *Am J Psychiatry* 136:79–83, 1979.

3. Chouinard G, de Montigny C, Annable L: Tardive dyskinesia and antiparkinsonian medication. *Am J Psychiatry* 136:228–229, 1979.

4. Christensen AV, Nielson IM: Dopaminergic supersensitivity: Influence of dopamine agonists, cholinergics, anticholinergics, and drugs used for the treatment of tardive dyskinesia. *Psychopharmacology* 62:111–116, 1979.

5. Hogarty GE, Schooler NR, Ulrich R, et al: Fluphenazine and social therapy in the aftercare of schizophrenic patients. *Arch Gen Psychiatry* 36:1283–1294, 1979.

6. Jellinek T, Gardos G, Cole JO: *Adverse Effects of Antiparkinsonian Drug Withdrawal.* 133rd Annual Meeting of the American Psychiatric Association, May, 1980.

7. Chouinard G, Annable L, Ross-Chouinard A: Comparison of fluphenazine esters in the treatment of schizophrenic outpatients: Extrapyramidal symptoms and therapeutic effect. *Am J Psychiatry* (in press).

15

Ethics and Tardive Dyskinesia

Panel Discussion

Robert W. Daly
Daniel E. Casey
Joseph DeVeaugh-Geiss
George E. Crane
Irwin Birnbaum
Bruce Dearing

The Psychiatrist as Moral Agent

Reflection on the kinds of moral problems that emerge from the practice of psychiatry can be remotely helpful to the psychiatrist and the patient in their resolution of the actual moral dilemmas and conflicts they experience. My reflections and recommendations pertinent to the resolution of the moral problems experienced by psychiatrists who treat psychotic patients with neuroleptic drugs are intended to be helpful in that way.

I. *There is a difference between technical problems and moral problems in psychiatry.*

Psychiatrists do their work without giving much thought to the morality of their acts because their attention is ordinarily directed at doing their work in a technically correct way. This habit is reinforced by clinical practice and the canons of scientific inquiry. Thus, when someone claims that this or that practice is "immoral," psychiatrists are prone to behave like fish who do not notice that they live in water until they are removed from it. When accused of immorality, many psychiatrists become angry and confused, and respond by saying, "No! Psychiatry is one thing, morality another!" — and then proceed to diagnose or to psychoanalyze their critics. This know-nothing approach or the know-everything approach (that identifies the whole of psychiatry with the whole of morality) to the problems of morality in psychiatry does not help us, our patients, or our critics. Everyone would be better served by a know-something approach.

The *first* thing the psychiatrist needs to know is the difference between a moral problem and a technical problem in psychiatry. Technical problems concern the means to an end. Do the ovens at the bakery — or at Dachau — work well? This kind of question is concerned with the efficacy, efficiency, complexity, or precision of an instrument, or a machine, or a performance in which a special skill is displayed. Inquiries of this kind are formulated as if there were no moral problems about the end itself, or about the connection between the means and the ends, or as if there were no moral conflicts concerning what human agents ought to do or to be. Is it well or good — in a moral sense — to work the ovens? A question of this sort is concerned with ends and with the activities of human agents insofar as they succeed or fail to respond to the fact that the sort of freedom one has as a human agent depends in part on the intentions of other agents.[1]

II. *Psychiatry is the moral institution which aims at the restoration, maintenance, or improvement of the sanity of particular human agents.*

Psychiatrists contend that psychiatry is one thing, morality another — especially when they are treating persons who are manifestly psychotic. Because the patient's infirmity is profound and summons the psychiatrist to his work in a clear and unproblematic way, the psychiatrist experiences the technical problems inherent in the treatment of the case as paramount. As a result, the moral dimension of the situation goes unnoticed. The *second* thing the psychiatrist needs to know (even when he is treating psychotic patients) is that he is engaged in an enterprise with a special moral aim. Consider why his activities are informed by a moral aim which is an essential, not simply incidental, characteristic of his work.

Madness deprives one, to a greater or lesser extent, of the ability to remain alive, to live, or to live well. Such a state acquires moral meaning because it constitutes a relative absence or negation of sanity. Sanity is the form of health that one enjoys when his behavior and experience are integrated with his knowledge and capacity to choose, so that he can, in *this* way, conduct himself as a human agent.

The effort — the psychiatrist's effort — to restore the patient to sanity is a special moral undertaking, because the freedom of action that is conferred by sanity and enjoyed by one person depends in part on what another person, the psychiatrist, does in the relationship. The psychiatrist has a special moral obligation in the relationship with the patient. It is to aid the patient in his attempt to restore or maintain his sanity. If the psychiatrist does not attend to this dimension of his work, the patient and others, if they are dissatisfied with the patient's progress, will remind him of it. Their complaints will indicate that psychiatry has this special moral aim and that it is, from an historical and social point of view, a moral institution. The psychiatrist should attend to these complaints and claims. He should recognize that it is reasonable to characterize his activities as morally right or wrong, even when he does not agree with the exact content of these claims.

What elements of morality should a psychiatrist display in a relationship with a patient in addition to attempting to restore the patient to sanity?

Like other professionals who have comparatively clear roles to play in the moral economy of the community, psychiatrists would prefer to learn about the general, as well as the special, morality of their office by being praised for their moral virtues and heroic deeds. But the truth of the matter is that one usually learns about the morality of the psychiatrist by hearing of the ways in which he is immoral. From a list of putative moral failings one can discern what is ordinarily expected of the psychiatrist from a moral point of view. For instance, it is said that the psychiatrist does not obey general moral rules (promise-keeping, truth-telling, respect for other people); that he acts for the wrong end (to secure wealth, the tranquility of the family or the hospital staff, the satisfaction of his sexual appetite, or the power to direct the lives of others); that he is too preoccupied with his problems to pay attention to the problems of his patient; that he lacks the requisite information or skills; that he makes errors of judgment; and that he lacks the virtue of understanding his place as a psychiatrist in the larger community. So, by implication, the psychiatrist should follow general moral rules, act for the right end in a competent manner, and know the place of his art and his office in that community. There is, in addition, a further expectation, one which is at the center of our concerns today. The psychiatrist, like other healers, should "do no harm."[2]

III. *A means to an end takes on moral significance in proportion to the moral significance of the end to which it is a means — and in proportion to the moral significance of whatever is known to occur or to be likely to occur as a consequence of employing that means.*

If what I have said so far is correct, then it should be apparent that the justification, when there is one, for prescribing neuroleptics turns on the specific form and value of sanity in the life of the patient and the actual place which neuroleptics are known to have in bringing about this state. There are, of course, many considerations to be taken into account when deciding what is to be done in an actual case, including considerations unique to that case. But we are primarily concerned with the moral meaning of the statistical knowledge indicating whether or not the use of neuroleptics *is* a means to sanity. The question in its general form can be put this way: given that the aim of the psychiatrist is to secure the sanity of patients who are psychotic, is it better with respect to *this* aim to prescribe neuroleptics (alone or in combination with other types of treatment) or to do nothing aside from general care, or to do something else? If neuroleptics were not a means to this end or were clearly an inferior* means compared with some other, there could be little justification for their employment, and moral difficulties occasioned by their use could be avoided. But the majority of investigators and clinicians hold that these drugs are a means to the end in some kinds of cases — though this opinion continues to be disputed. Clearly, from a statistical point of view, the efficacy of neuroleptics in the treatment of schizophrenia is not as great as that of the use of penicillin in the treatment of pneumococcal pneumonia.

So we are forced to consider the second part of proposition III. What else of moral significance is likely to occur as a consequence of using neuroleptics for the treatment of persons who are psychotic? Clinical research and clinical experience indicate that a considerable number and range of harms (and so the risks of these harms) can follow upon the use of neuroleptics. Hence, one finds a list of "side effects," "adverse reactions" (including tardive dyskinesia), "complications," "contraindications," and an attendant set of "warnings" and "cautions" associated with the use of these drugs. The moral questions before the psychiatrist and the patient are these: What is the moral worth of the patient's sanity? and, Is it worth suffering the risk of the harms, and possibly the harms as well, occasioned by the use of these drugs in order to secure benefits that neuroleptics may — or may not — in any particular case confer?

Because the good sought is highly esteemed and the dangers to be avoided are properly feared, and because the psychiatrist must presently choose to prescribe and the patient to take neuroleptics — or not — the wager for most people turns upon what is known about the likelihood of securing the benefits and avoiding the detriments. It is just at this point that clinical knowledge, or more correctly, the lack of such knowledge

---

*A treatment may be "inferior" in several ways: efficacious in a smaller percentage of cases, or less efficacious in every case, or associated with many more harms, etc, compared with some other treatment.

contributes to the creation of a moral dilemma. It is often difficult for the psychiatrist to make an unequivocal recommendation regarding the use of neuroleptics, based on statistical findings regarding benefits, harms, and risks. The frequency and duration of the benefits are not so great, nor are the harms so infrequent, transient, and trivial that one can in conscience proceed to employ neuroleptics as a standard therapy for certain classes of psychoses. But neither are the benefits so ephemeral and infrequent nor the risks so great that one can say, in conscience, that the use of these drugs cannot be recommended in many cases. That is one reason why the benefit/detriment/risk ratios must be carefully weighed in each case by the psychiatrist and the patient or his intimates (for it is the patient who suffers the risks and experiences the harms should they occur).

When the question about treatment with neuroleptics arises, both parties should recognize that:

They are cooperating under conditions of uncertainty;

The use of neuroleptics entails the possibility of irreparable, irreversible harms;

The denial or refusal of their use forecloses the possibility of a benefit which might not otherwise ensue — the mitigation of some or many features of the psychosis; and

The harms which may follow consequent to the use of neuroleptics or from the denial or refusal of their use do not constitute a wrong if informed consent is given by the patient or his intimates and due care is exercised in the provision of treatment by the psychiatrist.

If these and the other moral precepts I have mentioned are followed, neither party should fear moral blame from any quarter. Indeed, I would consider praising both parties — though the patient more than the psychiatrist — for proceeding with whatever decision is made. Either decision requires some measure of moral courage.

The form and content of a decision regarding the use of neuroleptics in the treatment of the psychoses is, after all, like many other decisions in medicine and in life. One often proceeds to make important decisions under conditions of uncertainty, knowing that no matter what he decides, harms as well as benefits may ensue. Some of these can be foreseen as possibilities, and some not. That is the *third* thing the psychiatrist needs to know.

Robert W. Daly

184

REFERENCES

1. Macmurray J: *Persons in Relation.* London, Faber and Faber, Ltd, 1961, p 119.
2. Jonsen AR: Do no harm: Axiom of medical ethics, in Spicker SF, Engelhardt T Jr (eds): *Philosophical Medical Ethics: Its Nature and Significance.* Dordrecht, Holland, D. Reidel Publishing Co, 1977, pp 27–46.

*　　　*　　　*　　　*

Treatment of Psychosis and Risk for Tardive Dyskinesia: The Risk Benefit Ratio

The problem of treating psychosis — the potential benefits *vs* the potential risks — or perhaps what has just been described as the detriment/benefit ratio, cannot be solved solely with a mathematical formula. We use the concept "ratio" to imply that we can accurately estimate the numbers involved. However, it is quite obvious that the solutions are not at all clear.

Some general principles can be offered to guide treatment decisions. When a psychotic patient is evaluated, a clinical choice must be made. It is a decision to treat or not to treat. There are substantial risks to no treatment, as patients with schizophrenia have more disrupted lives and higher suicide rates than the general population. On the other hand, there are risks of treatment to be balanced against the potential benefits. To rephrase the question, is neuroleptic treatment efficacious, and will the patient benefit? Antipsychotic drug treatment very effectively controls acute psychotic symptoms in the majority of schizophrenic patients. Neuroleptics are also effective, though somewhat less so, for maintaining symptom control in patients who benefited from drug treatment. Psychosocial interventions supplement pharmacological approaches and should be emphasized in patients who do not benefit from drug therapy. Relapse rates for patients successfully treated with neuroleptics and then transferred to placebo are significantly higher than for patients who are maintained on neuroleptics. Some patients who discontinue medications will not relapse, however, suggesting prolonged treatment is not required for everyone. The implication, then, is that the patients' needs may change later in treatment. A fixed, rigid approach to all clinical situations will lead to problems for the patient or the physician, or possibly for both. Patients do not stay the same over time, and neither should treatment approaches.

In summary, the relevant issues are: who is being treated, for what symptoms, with what drug and dose, for how long, and with what benefit? Successfully managing chronic psychiatric illness requires periodic reassessment and flexible treatment plans tailored to the individual needs of each patient.

Daniel E. Casey

*   *   *   *

Informed Consent for Neuroleptic Therapy

Considering the reported high incidence and prevalence rates for tardive dyskinesia (see Chapters 3 and 4), it seems apparent that the risk factor is significant for patients taking neuroleptic drugs. In addition, taking into consideration Doctor Daly's comments on the benefit/detriment equation, and keeping in mind the obvious physical and social disabilities imposed by the presence of abnormal involuntary movements, the development of dyskinesia as a complication of drug therapy becomes a very serious matter. The likelihood that the syndrome will be irreversible and the lack of any treatment for this condition place the treating physician and the patient at high risk for undesirable consequences. Therefore, both from the physician's point of view (perhaps defensively, to protect himself or herself from litigation), as well as from the patient's point of view — to protect the patient from harm, or at least to allow him or her to participate in judgments about risky procedures — informed consent would seem to be essential. Of course, informed consent should be obtained for all treatments, but specifically the risk of movement disorders ought to be mentioned when obtaining consent from patients who will receive neuroleptic drugs.

Table 15-1 shows the three essential elements of informed consent, and if one keeps these things in mind, one will at least obtain proper informed consent. The first element is that it must be voluntary. There cannot be any coercion, nor any condition that would make the patient feel he or she is obligated to give consent. What this really means is the patient must be willing of his or her own volition to take the treatment; he or she cannot be an involuntary psychiatric patient, for example, and give informed consent. The patient must be competent in order to receive the information. Competency is actually a legal matter but it is quasi-medical in the sense that the kinds of judgments that are made about competency often relate to diseases of the nervous system, and physicians make these kinds of medical judgments. But competency itself is a legal decision and might be made by the courts. And, finally, there must be information, and this is why it is called *informed* consent. Information should include a statement about what is being treated. Although Table 15-1 shows the word "diagnosis," it is not necessary to use the diagnosis proper, but simply to tell the patient what you are treating, or intend to treat, by the prescription of the neuroleptic. The patient should be told about available treatments, whatever these may be. In psychiatric practice, there are frequently few options, but the patient should be advised of them. Mention should be made of the risks and benefits of these other treatments, as well as the risks and benefits of the treatment proposed. The risks and benefits of no treatment, an option which is frequently overlooked, should be discussed with the patient, ie, the probable outcome if the patient does not receive treatment. Some people might choose no treatment if this were discussed. And it is necessary to disclose all risks of any significance. Insignificant risks do not require disclosure. A precedent established in malpractice litigation is that any risk with 3% or greater frequency of occurrence associated with a procedure is considered to be significant and requires disclosure.[1]

Table 15-1
Elements of Informed Consent

1. Voluntary
2. Competency (to be informed)
3. Information
   Diagnosis
   Available treatments
   Risks/benefits of treatments
   Risks/benefits of no treatment
   Must disclose all significant risks

Figure 15-1 is a flow chart which I have prepared to provide a model for the consent procedure. It shows two categories, the voluntary and the involuntary patient, according to the patient's status in the hospital. In my opinion, the involuntary patient cannot give consent and there is no need to think further about this, but it is probably advisable in such cases to obtain proxy consent, from a legal guardian, or relative, or family member. Among the voluntary patients, there are again two categories, the competent and the incompetent patient. The competent patient, after having a discussion with the physician about the treatment, will either consent in which case treatment proceeds, or will refuse to consent in which case treatment is withheld, as long as the patient is competent. The figure contains a line connecting the "no consent" box with the "incompetent" box, a line which I refer to as "catch-22." I am sure that I, as well as others, have seen this, and that is, if a patient who is considered to be competent does not consent to a treatment that we think will help and which we are sure is a good treatment, then there must be something wrong with him; I have seen people then declared incompetent, apparently because they did not consent. I do not recommend this but have included it in the figure for the sake of completeness. However, there should be no treatment if the patient does not give consent.

The incompetent patient, on the other hand, may be treated under a number of different models. A reasonable model, and for which there is certainly precedent, is the model of the comatose patient — a person with an acute neurologic injury that renders him incompetent. This is represented on the figure as the acute condition. In this case, the comatose patient is routinely treated without consent. I have broken this down further because in psychiatric practice our patients may not be unconscious and yet we may believe that they have an acute brain disease, or dysfunction, such as delirium. If the patient does not protest, then, in my opinion, he fits the model of the comatose patient. And, if he does not protest, then it is reasonable to proceed with treatment, even without consent. However, if the patient protests, then a somewhat different situation is faced than with the nonprotesting patient with acute brain dysfunction. In this instance, when a patient says he does not want the treatment, one should not, therefore, presume to treat such a patient without first obtaining proxy consent. This situation, that of the protesting incompetent patient, resembles that of the involuntary patient, a situation in which I do not believe informed consent is possible. The nonprotesting incompetent patient, on the other hand, may be treated without consent under this model.

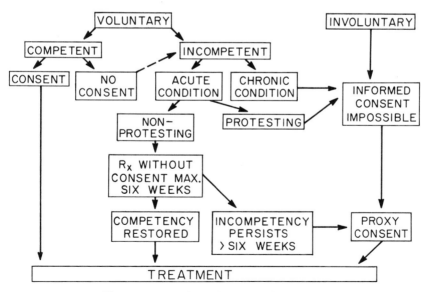

Figure 15-1 Informed consent flow chart.

In the model of the comatose patient who is unable to give consent for treatment while unconscious, the physician's ethical responsibility is to restore the patient to consciousness and competency, if possible, and then to obtain consent for further treatment. Once competency has been restored, the patient falls under the category of the voluntary, competent patient and enjoys the right to accept or refuse treatment. With the psychiatric patient being treated with neuroleptic drugs, and who is considered incompetent by virtue of psychosis, this model may apply and, once restored to competency, the patient should be asked for consent for further treatment. My arbitrary guideline, as outlined in Figure 15-1, is to treat without consent for a maximum of six weeks, for the following reasons: 1) I have seen tardive dyskinesia develop within six weeks from the initiation of neuroleptic therapy, although this is quite uncommon — usually tardive dyskinesia occurs after a year or two or more of therapy. However, I think that the risk for tardive dyskinesia is truly negligible during the first six weeks of therapy, and that this can be considered a safe period; and 2) most neuroleptic therapies, if they are going to be effective, will be so by the time that six weeks have elapsed, and if they are not by that time, they are likely to still not be effective six months later. So, this is a reasonably good arbitrary cutoff point. And, at the sixth week of therapy, assuming the patient has an acute dysfunction that is treatable, then competency might be restored. If the incompetency persists for more than six weeks, then we are treating a patient with a chronic condition that renders him incompetent, and there may be reason to expect no significant change in that condition in the foreseeable future. This situation leads to the necessity for proxy consent as would be obtained with the involuntary patients.

In summary, there is only one condition that permits informed consent and that is of the voluntary, competent patient. I recommend obtaining proxy consent for involuntary patients, for incompetent patients with chronic conditions, and for incompetent patients with acute conditions if they are protesting the treatment. Within this model, I see treatment without consent as permissible only for the patient with an acute condition that renders him incompetent, who does not protest, for whom treatment may restore competency, and for no more than six weeks. If, after six weeks, competency is restored, then voluntary informed consent for further treatment should be obtained from the patient. If competency is not restored during this time, then proxy consent is recommended.

Joseph DeVeaugh-Geiss

REFERENCE

1. Louisell DW, Williams H: *Medical Malpractice, vol 2.* New York, Matthew Bender, 1975, p 594.47.

*   *   *   *

Medical and Legal Responsibilities
of Physicians Prescribing Neuroleptics

Who is responsible for tardive dyskinesia which now afflicts thousands of persons? Suppose a patient experiences his first episode of schizophrenia and Doctor A treats him with a neuroleptic with some success and no significant ill effects. Doctor A can truthfully say: "My patient has not had any problem while under my care; I cannot be held responsible for what may happen to him later on." Suppose that the same patient relapses several times over the next 10 or 20 years and is treated by Doctors B, C, D, and E who administer one or more neuroleptic drugs. Finally, Doctor F discovers that his patient has unmistakable signs of tardive dyskinesia while he is receiving chemotherapy. Doctor F may have some justification when he explains to his patient or family that tardive dyskinesia is the result of the cumulative effects of drug therapy. Hence, he cannot be held responsible for all the drugs prescribed by other physicians. Now our patient has a psychosis as well as tardive dyskinesia. He must be admitted to a hospital and is placed under the care of Doctor G who immediately orders intensive chemotherapy. He reasons that the patient is disturbed and the only available therapy is the intensive use of psychotropic drugs. It may aggravate the motor abnormalities of the tongue and jaw and even cause a life-threatening dysphagia. On the other hand, it is not Doctor G's fault if the patient received so much medication from Doctors A, B, C, etc.

One may question the innocence of the practitioners, but others must be held responsible for the misery of so many patients who have been treated with the neuroleptics. Doctors write the orders, but the marketing of drugs is done by industry. President Coolidge once said: "The business of America is business." Since we live in the same capitalistic system, the business of the drug companies is business. This does not mean that the sale of a product cannot benefit humanity and, at the same time, be a source of income for the shareholders. On the other hand, certain features that endanger the safety of the consumer will reduce the marketability of the product, hence all industries, including drug companies, will ignore the problem as long as possible. In 1968, the evidence that tardive dyskinesia was a common side effect of all neuroleptics was overwhelming, yet it was not until 1972 or 1973 that drug companies included adequate information on tardive dyskinesia in the package inserts of their neuroleptic drugs. Academia, the FDA, and the NIMH have also been slow in recognizing the magnitude of the problem.

Recently, the literature on tardive dyskinesia has increased exponentially and a considerable amount of research is carried out in hospitals and in the laboratories. Yet the practice of drug use has changed little, at least in my experience. Physicians may be blamed for not familiarizing themselves with the more recent advances in this field, but the information they may obtain from scientific publications are not always very helpful. Physicians are advised to prescribe medication in doses that are both effective and nonhazardous. But how can a practitioner decide which one is the dose that benefits his patient?

Schizophrenia (and most other mental diseases) has an unpredictable course; besides, the assessment of what constitutes real improvement is one of the most controversial issues in psychiatry. Even the most systematic studies utilizing rating scales, double blind techniques, and random assignment to therapeutic modalities are not successful in establishing optimal treatment regimens. As for the safety of dose levels, the problem is even more formidable, because the long term effects of neuroleptics are insidious and unpredictable in individual cases. Thus, the advice to use the minimum of chemotherapy that is effective and safe is at best gratuitous. Efforts to find a cure for tardive dyskinesia have not yet reached the point where they can help the practicing physician. The many drugs screened for the purpose of reducing motor disabilities have been ineffective or are still in the experimental stage. Thus, the psychiatrist can only hope that the patient treated with neuroleptics will get better and will not develop permanent dyksinesias.

Hospitalization for the refractory psychotic patient may be an alternative. There is no doubt that a substantial proportion of schizophrenics become more psychotic when the use of chemotherapy is discontinued, but not all persons who no longer receive drugs become murderers, arsonists or rapists. Usually, the patient's condition becomes more precarious and may cause unacceptable hardship to his family or the community. Such patients could be effectively handled without chemotherapy in a hospital or in a facility that has the function of a hospital, but is called something else. This alternative, however, is unthinkable in the 25th year of community-oriented psychiatry.

In the first place, there are not sufficient beds in hospitals for the mentally ill and most institutions do not have rational programs for the care of the chronic patient. Second, the psychiatric profession and society in general are firmly convinced that hospitalization is a failure and must be used only as the last resort. (In many clinical studies, rehospitalization or time spent in an institution is a criterion measure for the effectiveness of a treatment procedure.) Most psychiatrists think that all schizophrenics must receive chemotherapy. If the results are unsatisfactory, doses are increased; and if this does not work, another neuroleptic is prescribed. In the event the hospital has a research unit for the screening of investigational new drugs, the patient is included in a research program. It does not occur to the physician that the use of neuroleptics is not the right therapy for many mentally ill people (see also Chapter 14).

Current practices of drug use by the psychiatric profession cannot be defended, but one cannot ignore the role played by economic, social, and political forces.

George E. Crane

*   *   *   *

Tardive Dyskinesia — Medico-Legal Considerations

In assessing the benefits of neuroleptic medication, and how society deals with them, I would like to quote from the remarks of the Assistant Director of the Illinois Department of Corrections concerning the use of fluphenazine (Prolixin) and chlorpromazine (Thorazine) on inmates in the Illinois prison system. "Such drugs," he says, "are more effective and humane than man-handling or shackles." Now I think that expresses the attitude of some members of the public toward the use of neuroelptic medication. This makes me wonder about the attitudes of some members of our profession, the law and medicine, concerning the use of neuroleptic medication in prisons as a substitute for man-handling and shackles. Moreover, I wonder how often neuroleptic drugs are prescribed today in mental hospitals as a substitute for man-handling and shackles, or as a surrogate for a form of organic somatic treatment that previously served as a substitute for man-handling and shackles. It is in this area, where neuroleptic medications are used to control behavior in both prisons and hospitals, that the law, and more particularly, the interdisciplinary relationship of law and medicine, has been most deficient in helping people.

As you may already know, the common law is an adversary process where lawyers appear in opposing positions in the courtroom for their clients. An essential element of the adversary process is that the lawyer, by necessity, must analyze the situation before him in a pragmatic and cynical fashion. I think that the use of neuroleptic medications should also be analyzed in terms of the pragmatic and cynical approach that lawyers customarily take. Then, perhaps, the rights and needs of the patient would be adequately represented in the decision as to whether to prescribe neuroleptic medications.

For lawyers specializing in malpractice litigation, one of the problems frequently confronted is the irresponsibility of physicians in the courtroom. I am referring to physicians who either appear in the courtroom in an irresponsible manner or refuse to appear in the courtroom *at all* in an irresponsible manner. What do I mean by those who fail to appear and thus act in an irresponsible manner? As you already know, it is sometimes difficult to locate people with both knowledge and respectability to appear as witnesses in medical malpractice cases. This has led to a situation at the bar in which we have a group of lawyers who characteristically appear as patients' counsel and another group of lawyers who characteristically appear as physicians' counsel. Furthermore, the insurance companies who insure physicians will not allow them to be represented by lawyers who frequently appear as patients' counsel. In these cases, lawyers find that respected and learned physicians will not come forward to testify in malpractice cases. This is because physicians are frequently *so* self-indoctrinated or institutionalized with the idea of being "Doctors" that often they will not do anything which they feel would harm a colleague. Since respectable physicians will not *always* come forward to testify in medical malpractice cases, frequently irresponsible physicians, who will testify to anything, do come forward to testify in those cases. This background must be given some thought before we consider, any further, the use of neuroleptic medication.

When we talk about risk/benefit ratios in anything, we must ask, as Doctor Daly so correctly pointed out, whose benefit are we serving? This is especially true in psychiatry. Society is not quite ready yet to embrace the saying: "Tarry not his ghost, oh let him pass. He hates him that would upon the rack of this tough world, stretch him out longer." That statement comes from the master psychologist in *King Lear*. Yet, when we prevent the suicide, whose benefit are we serving? New York State, in an action for wrongful death — which simply means that the death of a person is caused by another person's carelessness or negligence — allows damages only for pecuniary loss. Pecuniary loss is defined as the support and services which the people who were dependent upon the decedent could reasonably have expected to receive from the decedent if he or she had lived. Therefore, saving a person from being stretched longer on the rack of this tough world really only benefits those people who could look to that person for support. Neither the law nor medicine is prepared to confront that situation. As a lawyer, looking at this situation from the cynical perspective of the adversary in the courtroom, I would have to say that as a physician you must always opt for life or you may be held responsible.

Let us turn now to the statements Doctor Casey made. What he was saying, in legal terms, was that the use of neuroleptic medication is a matter of medical judgment. As you already know, a physician cannot be held liable for a mere error in judgment. That is the law. However, the law also says that a physician cannot be held liable for a mere error in judgment, provided he has first made a careful examination of the patient and provided that he or she has the necessary information upon which to base that judgment. In my pro forma case, the physician saw the patient on a six months' basis, but only to ask the patient, "How are you getting along?" The patient said, "Fine," and the physician renewed her prescription. The failure to look for facial grimacing, tremor, worm-like movements of the tongue, lip pursing, or other signs of incipient tardive dyskinesia, is the error for which the physician will be held liable. *"How are you getting along?" is not a careful examination.*

In considering the doctrine of consent and its relationship to tardive dyskinesia, it has now become a relatively simple problem because we now have established the criteria for the kind of information that must be given to a patient prior to the administration of neuroleptic medication. I have made available some excerpts from the opinion of the United States Court of Appeals for the District of Columbia Circuit in Canterbury *v* Spence. In that case, the court held that the patient should be informed of all of the inherent risks in the contemplated treatment that a reasonably prudent person in the patient's position would expect to be informed of. Unfortunately, that is not the law in New York. New York State has, at the request of the New York State Medical Society, codified the law of informed consent. Until July of 1975, a physician who proposed to perform an operation, a diagnostic procedure, or a treatment, was under a duty to make an understandable disclosure to the patient. He was required to explain to the patient what he proposed to do and to explain, in terms understandable by a reasonable person, the reason for the procedure and its inherent risks.

Today, the New York law requires that a physician before performing an operation, a diagnostic procedure, or treatment is under a duty to explain to the patient, in understandable terms, the nature of the proposed procedure, the risks and benefits of the procedure, and the alternative procedures available. The physician has a duty to explain to the patient all the facts that a reasonable medical practitioner would explain, so that the patient may give his consent to the procedure with an awareness of: 1) his existing condition; 2) the purpose of, and the advantage of submitting to the procedure, and the risks to the patient's health or life that the procedure may impose; 3) the risks involved if no treatment is given; and 4) the available alternative procedures and the risks and advantages involved in them. I want to note with great particularity, in regard to the codification of the New York law, that what I have read is the suggested language in what is known as New York State's *Pattern Jury Instructions*. It is a book of proposed jury instructions, which the judicial conference of the state suggests that the trial judge read to the jury. Although it does not mean that each trial judge will follow those particular instructions word for word, they are essentially what is required in New York.

Psychiatry is not the only medical specialty with problems of informed consent. I would like to read to you the consent form used by a regional hospital in a request for sterilization. It says, "We (the husband and wife both sign) being of sound mind, request that Doctor "X" and assistants of his choice perform upon Mrs. "Y" the following operation: Bilateral, partial salpingectomy." However, this patient was not going to have a bilateral salpingectomy. This patient was going to have a "tubelication." If you do not know what a "tubelication" is, you should know that most of the clients who come to see me, as a result of some error in performing a tubal ligation, believe that they are having a "tubelication" and that they have no idea what a "salpingectomy" is. We might all be better off if we referred to it as "tubelication," instead of tubal ligation, because then the doctors and the patients would be talking about the same thing, or at least, to paraphrase Lewis Carroll: "Every word I use, means whatever I choose it to mean." These patients think that they are going to have their tubes tied. *Some know what the tubes are and some do not.* Nevertheless, they are going to have their tubes tied. In many cases, the patient has been on the witness stand being questioned by the attorney for the physician, and she is totally confused as to whether she was supposed to become sterile or she was supposed to become fertile. That is "informed consent." Furthermore, this hospital form goes on to say, "It has been explained to us that this operation is intended to result in sterility, although this result has not been guaranteed. We understand that a sterile person is not capable of becoming a parent." Apparently, adoption is not open to sterile persons. It further states: "We voluntarily request the operation and understand that if it proves successful, the results will be permanent. It will thereafter be physically impossible for the patient to inseminate or to conceive or to bear children." How she was going to inseminate in the first place, I do not know. Finally, it states: "We do hereby release the attending physician, Doctor "X" and "Z" Hospital from any claims and/or responsibilities of the performance of such operation."

Well, now for whose benefit was this informed consent written? The tragedy, however, of this particular case was that this patient was not advised of the mortality rate of sterilization by laparoscopy, which has been reported at 0.3%. Perhaps patients would choose some other form of contraception rather than risk a 0.3% mortality rate and the higher morbidity rate. The patient was not advised that in 1 out of 300 laparoscopy ligations, the iliac artery on one side or the other is lacerated. In this particular case, the obstetrician/gynecologist lacerated the abdominal aorta. When the patient lost her blood pressure, the physician called for the CPR team, but the patient died.

If this patient was entitled to more information, can we say that any other patient is entitled to any less information when there is any risk of morbidity or mortality involved in the proposed treatment? I ask you, who is to decide? Until we answer that question, the courts and the legislatures will determine who is to decide. We must look at questions involving informed consent in malpractice litigation, not in terms of who will prevail and what are the risk/benefit ratios to the patient and the physician, but in terms of its role in society and, especially, if we are involved in the specialty of psychiatry, which is concerned with behavior patterns that are unacceptable to society.

In conclusion, I would like to make reference to one of Doctor Crane's articles in which he said that he had been to one institution and had surveyed it to determine how much neuroleptic medication they were using. Afterward, he talked to them about the dangers of prescribing high dosages of medications as a form of treatment for chronically institutionalized patients. However, when he returned to the institution six months later, the psychiatrists were prescribing the same amounts of neuroleptic medication. Doctor Crane had written about the dangers of neuroleptic medication, he had talked about it, and still no one was really listening, at least, not the physicians at that institution. And he asked: "What good is it for us to do this if no one will listen?" Well, maybe, litigation will have the effect of making physicians listen under these circumstances.

Irwin Birnbaum

*   *   *   *

Patient Perspectives on Iatrogenic Disease

Most of what I can contribute will be interpretations and observations from a lay point of view, not precisely as a patient advocate, but as an interested witness relying on projection and introspection, rather than on laboratory data. There are three points that I would like to make about what might be called the social meaning of dyskinesia or movement disorders. The first concerns the perception by ordinary people of those afflicted by movement disorders; the second concerns the self-perception of a patient with tardive dyskinesia; and the third comprehends practical, defensive considerations as well as moral imperatives in calculation of risk/benefit in administering psychotropic drugs, taking into account the psychosocial interaction of the physician, the institution, the family, and all those concerned with the patient, as well as the patient himself.

We need only to glance at history to reflect on the cruelties inflicted in the Middle Ages on the victims of St. Vitus' dance. We wince at the identification of sufferers as being in league with the devil, or being afflicted with demonic tendencies on the evidence of certain kinds of movement disorders, particularly as related to facial grimaces. The haunting story of the Pied Piper of Hamelin evokes the principle of punishment or vengeance through movement disorders. Similarly in the very grim, Grimm's fairy tale of the *Red Shoes,* the little girl was punished for her pride by being locked into the red shoes which danced her into exhaustion and on to her death. In the arresting play *Marat & Sade,* set in a madhouse, the playwright, the director, and the actors have made powerfully effective use of movement disorders as a means of portraying and commenting upon madness, evoking the laughter and terror of comedy, rather than the pity and terror of tragedy. For characters in that play, movement disorders serve to define individual madness and alienation from the rest of the world.

If we focus upon the movement disorders most closely related to tardive dyskinesia — movements of the tongue and the mouth — one reflects on the way in which the gargoyles decorating countless cathedrals are presented: most of them have hideous faces with tongues protruding. In many cultures, thrusting out the tongue is recognized as a term of derision, of insult, even of obscenity, and in many circumstances considered an embarrassing sexual provocation. In Ken Kesey's play *One Flew over the Cuckoo's Nest* (he being no friend to psychiatry or especially to institutionalization of the psychiatric patient), we may remember that in the initial encounter which sets McMurphy on a collision course with Big Nurse Ratched (who ultimately will have him lobotomized), he greets her impudently by darting his tongue at her in derision and raffish sexual provocation. The vulgar symbolization of retardation characteristically featuring the lolling tongue projects both fear and contempt, equating movement disorders of this kind with mental deficiencies quite inappropriately associated with many conditions ignorantly lumped together. I think, for example, of several persons with cerebral palsy who are regularly subjected to exquisite torture. Although they are high in intelligence, highly qualified professional people, taxpayers and contributors to the public weal, they often overhear themselves being referred to as "retards" because of the fact that they cannot control facial grimaces and movements of the tongue. On such evidence, it would seem that there are significant consequences of this particular kind of dyskinesia which could strongly affect a sensitive and sentient patient.

The second point is that those suffering from tardive dyskinesia sometimes perceive themselves differently. Doctor DeVeaugh-Geiss mentioned the denial on the part of some patients. I have observed patients who seem either unaware of, or unwilling to acknowledge, facial grimaces and lolling tongues unmistakably evident to all who were witnessing the persons. I am told that some people, particularly those with Huntington's chorea, at least affect indifference to what is happening within them and around them, and that the problem is perceived or structured as a difficulty for those who must relate to them. "I am behind my face; it is the one in the front who gets the jar," as the witticism goes. This, nevertheless, raises a serious question. If, by medical procedures, a paranoid fantasy (ie, that everyone is looking at me and regarding me with fear, contempt or revulsion) is supplanted by an objective situation in which that perception is fulfilled, a moral issue emerges. The first time I saw Doctor DeVeaugh-Geiss's remarkable film on tardive dyskinesia, I was immediately struck by the fact that in several of these scenes the patient was barefoot. I assume the purpose was to permit easy observation of movements in all the extremities. However, this triggered recollections of a stratagem sometimes employed by military interrogators of prisoners of war. It is apparently an exceedingly effective device for humiliating prisoners and breaking the will to resist, merely to force a POW always to appear barefoot when others are comfortably shod. It can be an assault on dignity and sense of self, whenever, in any significant way, one is caught, or compelled to remain "out of uniform." Recently a great deal of attention has been devoted to concerns of the individual selfhood and personal dignity of patients, with a recognition of the human costs of "depersonalization," "dehumanization," and excessive abstraction in relating to patients within the medical setting. Since, in our culture so much attention is given and significance attached to facial expression and body language, it would seem that side effects of therapeutic regimens need to be examined in a social context as well as a medical context, in terms of symbolic meaning as well as biochemical and physiological effect.

Finally, we may need to reflect upon a social movement of the past half century or so which has been called the "deauthorization of authority," institutional and personal. Our uneasiness about the aeronautical engineers who designed the engine mounts for the DC-10 leads to wondering what technical hazards lurk in 747s and other high technology artifacts. When we reflect that even though we are assured of back-ups for back-ups in protection against nuclear disaster, they did not work particularly well at Three Mile Island or in several other inadvertencies in the United States and abroad. The Watergate scandal is only the most dramatic of a variety of instances in which the unquestioned authority of government, of the church, of the university, and of the physician has gone by the board. There may be pressing reasons for taking cognizance of the social and psychological setting within which political and technical issues are being debated and decided.

Let us remind ourselves of the root meaning of "iatrogenic disease." *Iatros,* as I understand it, is the Greek word not for the physician, but for the place in which, in the Hippocratic era, medical treatment took place. Thus the "medical nemesis" of Ivan Ilych is not specifically *physician-induced* disorder, but is *treatment-induced* disorder. The dynamics of treatment really comprehends what the institution needs, what the physician needs, what the family needs. I do not know quite how to deal with this complexity, other than to confess that I have never been entirely easy with the parable of the shepherd who left the 90 and 9 unattended in order to range afield to retrieve that one last lost sheep. I wonder what would have happened had the wolves descended on the 90 and 9 in his absence. While instinctively I identify with what Doctor Crane was saying about the importance of remembering it is the patient we are serving, and not the family, and not our own needs; nonetheless all of our activity takes place in a social setting, which can complicate the issues.

Bruce Dearing

THE FIRST REPORT OF TARDIVE DYSKINESIA
IN PATIENTS TAKING NEUROLEPTIC DRUGS

Editor's Note: Chlorpromazine (Thorazine) was introduced into clinical practice in the early 1950s and, due to the impressive response shown by many patients receiving this drug, it was extensively used in Europe and the United States during that decade and subsequently. As would be expected with any side effect developing after chronic exposure to a drug, the syndrome of tardive dyskinesia was not recognized until many years after the introduction of chlorpromazine. The first known report, describing three cases, was published in German in 1957 in reply to a prior report which described what appeared to be acute dystonic reactions in patients taking chlorpromazine.

Although this report may be only of academic interest at this time, an English translation is provided as an appendix to this book for the curiosity of interested readers.

Beitrag zu der Mitteilung von Kulenkampff und Tarnow
Ein eigentumliches Syndrom im oralen Bereich bei Megaphenapplikation

(A Contribution to a Communication of Kulenkampff and Tarnow:
A Strange Syndrome in the Oral Area with Application of
Chlorpromazine)

Matthias Schonecker
Nervenarzt 28:35, 1957

The following case deviates, in spite of similarities, in some points from the phenomena earlier described.[1] An 18-year-old high school pupil [experienced a] first schizophrenic break three years ago. Because of a second attack with fearful agitation and compulsive washing [he was admitted for] hospital treatment. Because insulin and ECT were refused, the patient received 225 mg of chlorpromazine and 6 mg of reserpine daily. On the 12th day of treatment the patient looked up the writer in the afternoon. Because of right-sided stiffness the patient moved, helped by two fellow patients, hopping on the left leg. The lips were bent forward in "snout-cramp-position" and the muscles of the neck were tense. He could hardly talk intelligibly and complained of trouble breathing. The condition lasted approximately five minutes, subsided completely, and reappeared a half hour later. This time the patient lay in bed, pale and sweaty. [His] pulse was weak and frequent (140/minute) [and] there was an increased tone in the right extremities like rigor, without increased reflexes or focal signs of lesion of the pyramidal tracts. The tension and the "snout-cramp-position" were clearly present and the facial expression was anxious and labored. After injection of one ampoule of Effortil [a sympathomimetic amine] subcutaneously, the condition subsided ten minutes later. We also gave one ampoule of Depot Novadral [also a sympathomimetic amine] and chlorpromazine was immediately discontinued. During subsequent treatment with 4 to 6 mg reserpine this condition did not reappear. Neurologically, we could not find any abnormalities either before or after the attack. This observation is interesting in the respect that the cramps were not confined to the area of the cranial nerves and that the right-sided increase in tone was obviously of extrapyramidal origin.

We have observed oral automatisms with licking and smacking movements of the lips frequently in older (occasionally also younger) patients on chlorpromazine-reserpine medication which could have some connection with the above-described syndrome. These phenomena are mostly reversible after discontinuation of the medication. With three of our patients the syndrome continued for weeks and months until discharge.

1. Patient St, a 61-year-old female, [appearing] older than stated age, [with] whining melancholia. After eight weeks of chlorpromazine 225 mg daily [she developed] remarkable smacking movements of the lips that did not disappear after reduction to 75 to 100 mg daily in the following 12 weeks of treatment.

2. Patient M, a 66-year-old female [with] depression on the basis of cerebral sclerosis. After three weeks of treatment with chlorpromazine 200 mg (2 tid and 10 ml IM) and 6 mg reserpine daily [she developed a] pronounced parkinsonian syndrome and continuous licking of the lips. Chlorpromazine and reserpine were completely discontinued. After four weeks of biperiden, 2 tid, the parkinsonian syndrome was reduced to minimal residuals at discharge. The licking of the lips continued, however, as severely as before.

3. Patient K, a 62-year-old female, cerebral sclerotic, [in an] anxious and agitated condition. After 14 days of treatment with chlorpromazine 175 mg daily and reserpine 6 mg daily, both drugs were discontinued because of a developing parkinsonian syndrome. We later gave biperiden 1 tid. The smacking movements which had developed during the first days of treatment continued during the following 11 weeks of treatment until discharge.

In all three patients, a cerebral sclerosis [cerebral arteriosclerosis] was present. Patient K had minimal parkinsonian symptoms (mild tremor of one hand, lack of facial expressions) prior to treatment. Due to the continuous smacking movements, which were repulsive to other people and were voluntarily suppressible only for a short period of time, we could not avoid inflammation of the upper lip in spite of painstaking care. Patient St developed a furuncle of the upper lip.

ACKNOWLEDGMENT

The editor thanks Dr. Anselm George for assistance in translating from the German.

REFERENCE

1. Kulenkampff C, Tarnow G: Ein eigentumliches syndrom im oralen bereich bei megaphenapplikation. *Nervenarzt* 27:178–180, 1956.

THE ABNORMAL INVOLUNTARY MOVEMENT SCALE (AIMS)

Examination Procedure

Either before or after completing the Examination Procedure observe the patient unobtrusively, at rest (eg, in waiting room).

The chair to be used in this examination should be a hard, firm one without arms.

1. Ask patient whether there is anything in his/her mouth (ie, gum, candy, etc) and if there is, to remove it.

2. Ask patient about the *current* condition of his/her teeth. Ask patient if he/she wears dentures. Do teeth or dentures bother patient *now?*

3. Ask patient whether he/she notices any movements in mouth, face, hands, or feet. If yes, ask to describe and to what extent they *currently* bother patient or interfere with his/her activities.

4. Have patient sit in chair with hands on knees, legs slightly apart, and feet flat on floor. (Look at entire body for movements while in this position.)

5. Ask patient to sit with hands hanging unsupported. If male, between legs, if female and wearing a dress, hanging over knees. (Observe hands and other body areas.)

6. Ask patient to open mouth. (Observe tongue at rest within mouth.) Do this twice.

7. Ask patient to protrude tongue. (Observe abnormalities of tongue movement.) Do this twice.

8. Ask patient to tap thumb, with each finger, as rapidly as possible for 10–15 seconds; separately with right hand, then with left hand. (Observe facial and leg movements.)*

9. Flex and extend patient's left and right arms (one at a time). (Note any rigidity.)

10. Ask patient to stand up. (Observe in profile. Observe all body areas again, hips included.)

11. Ask patient to extend both arms outstretched in front with palms down. (Observe trunk, legs, and mouth.)*

12. Have patient walk a few paces, turn, and walk back to chair. (Observe hands and gait.) Do this twice.*

---

*Activated movements

ABNORMAL INVOLUNTARY MOVEMENT SCALE (AIMS)

Instructions

Complete examination procedure before making ratings.

Movement ratings Rate highest severity observed. Rate movements that occur upon activation one *less* than those observed spontaneously.

	(Circle One)*				
Facial and Oral Movements					
Muscles of Facial Expression eg, movements of forehead, eyebrows, periorbital area, cheeks; include frowning, blinking, smiling, grimacing	0	1	2	3	4
Lips and Perioral Area eg, puckering, pouting, smacking	0	1	2	3	4
Jaw eg, biting, clenching, chewing, mouth opening, lateral movement	0	1	2	3	4
Tongue Rate only increase in movement both and out mouth, NOT inability to sustain movement	0	1	2	3	4
Extremity Movements					
Upper *(arms, wrists, hands, fingers)* Include choreic movements (ie, rapid, objectively purposeless, irregular, spontaneous), athetoid movements (ie, slow, irregular, complex, serpentine). Do NOT include tremor (ie, repetitive, regular, rhythmic)	0	1	2	3	4
Lower *(legs, knees, ankles, toes)* eg, lateral knee movement, foot tapping, heel dropping, foot squirming, inversion and eversion of foot	0	1	2	3	4
Trunk Movements					
Neck, shoulders, hips eg, rocking, twisting, squirming, pelvic gyrations	0	1	2	3	4

Global Judgments		
Severity of abnormal movements	None, normal	0
	Minimal	1
	Mild	2
	Moderate	3
	Severe	4

Incapacitation due to abnormal movements	None, normal	0
	Minimal	1
	Mild	2
	Moderate	3
	Severe	4
Patient's awareness of abnormal movements	No awareness	0
Rate only patient's report	Aware, no distress	1
	Aware, mild distress	2
	Aware, moderate distress	3
	Aware, severe distress	4

Dental Status
Current problems with teeth and/or dentures	No	0
	Yes	1
Does patient usually wear dentures?	No	0
	Yes	1

*Code: 0 = None, 1 = Minimal, may be extreme normal, 2 = Mild, 3 = Moderate, 4 = Severe.